BABY CODES

101 Winning Combinations To Help Your Baby Sleep

Kevin Mills

MILLS Creative MINDS

MILLS Creative MINDS

PRAISE FOR BABY CODES

Every new parent I work with is worn out, sleep-deprived, and exhausted! They need quick, easy solutions to help their baby sleep through the night. Too many parents are running on empty and are unable to fully enjoy this special time. By reading **Baby Codes** you will quickly discover 101 unique, diverse and practical suggestions to help you relax, knowing you have lots of tried and tested solutions at your fingertips.

— SUE ATKINS, FOUNDER, POSITIVE-PARENTS.COM

Baby Codes is an organized, easy-to-read and humorous book of varied techniques to help your baby sleep. Whenever a sleepless parent needs help – *fast* – **Baby Codes** is ready and waiting with a quick tip to help get babies to sleep.

Baby Codes shines with creative tips for **all** parents —
new or experienced — on how to get their babies to
sleep. As a bonus, it's guaranteed to make even the most
sleep-deprived parent laugh (*or at least stop sobbing*).
Upon finishing it your first thought will be wondering
if Kevin Mills would be willing to move in to put your
newborn to sleep for you (*I asked him already. Sadly, he
kindly declined. For now.*) Your second thought will be to
question how anyone managed bedtime before **Baby
Codes** arrived.

With a sense of humor that can only come from
experience, Kevin Mills offers concise, easy-to-
understand advice for sleep-deprived parents. Based on
personal experience and extensive research, **Baby
Codes** is a full of creative ideas to get your kids to
sleep. As a father of five young boys, I have found **Baby
Codes** to be a great resource.

Baby Codes is one of those books you just have to have
around if you spend any time around babies. Old and

new ideas alike are sprinkled with humor and interesting facts. We all need to get our good night's sleep, and Kevin Mills gives some great tips on how to do just that!

This isn't your grandmother's baby book! As a busy mama of five, I thought I knew all the bedtime tricks for babies. **Baby Codes** is full of fresh remedies for exhausted parents. Easy-to-use with a nice dose of humor. I love it!

Baby Codes is an invaluable resource for anyone who has or cares for a baby. The tips are short, sweet and to the point. And there's a solution for every baby! Definitely a must-have on any parent's bookshelf!

Baby Codes is great! Very simple, useful tools that I have personally used and know for a matter-of-fact that they work. As a mother of two, I would highly recommend this book!

Having raised three children and spending many sleepless nights trying to get them to sleep, I wish I had had this book on my nightstand. I will definitely be giving **Baby Codes** to my two nieces who are expecting early next year. Maybe I can give them the greatest gift of all... SLEEP!

Kevin Mills presents a fresh (and fun!) approach to the time-worn problem of getting a baby to drift off to neverland. **Baby Codes** offers a comprehensive list of remedies, each concisely written for those parents who need assistance with getting their baby to sleep but do not have the time (or the desire) to read an exhaustive manual.

Kevin is onto something big with **Baby Codes**. As a weary mom, if I ever get a chance to read a book, it has to be quick and easy to follow because, let's face it, I can barely string five words together to make a complete sentence (*let alone read that same sentence*). You'll find yourself laughing out loud with Kevin's clever wit and sly confidence as he suggests code after code to use in deciphering your baby. **Baby Codes** is full of great, easy-to-use options that inspire hope that one day soon, you will sleep soundly. A refreshing resource for weary moms everywhere!

Sleep deprivation makes crazies of us all. Raising a newborn while working on 2 hrs sleep (a week) is sometimes a cruel reality! The humor and insight that **Baby Codes** offers during this insanity-inducing time is a welcome treat for any new mom!

You're a new parent, you're sleep deprived, and everyone keeps telling you babies "don't come with instruction manuals." Don't believe them. **Baby Codes is that elusive manual every parent is looking for.** Read it. Read it *now, (while you're still able to keep your eyes open)*.

As a mother of two, **Baby Codes is a godsend.** My first child? No sleep problems whatsoever. My second? She'd sleep for an hour or so. A day. **Baby Codes** is wonderful! (I only wish he would have written it sooner!) With so many techniques to offer, I'm confident **Baby Codes** will be around forever.

Baby Codes is beautifully organized, filled with

wonderful advice and laced with belly laughing humor. It's fun reading, even if you don't have kids! **Baby Codes is a must-have for all parents, grandparents and babysitters!** When you're stressed out trying to get the little one to sleep, you can't think of everything – but Kevin has, and he put it all in this amazing book. Loved It!!!

— DALETTE STOWELL, MOTHER OF 3, GRANDMOTHER OF 5

ACKNOWLEDGMENTS

I am not an island.

This book simply would not be in your hands if a handful of good people didn't donate their time, energy and insights to help make it happen. So as comprehensively as I can, I'm going to try to thank each and every single one of you.

To Kim: You are the wife every man hopes for. Your long-suffering patience, unconditional love and constant words of encouragement have meant the world to me. (Plus, you made three awesome kids, without whom I'd have had a seriously hard time writing this book.) I am a lucky, lucky man, and I love you dearly!

To Kyler, Kaleb & Kara: You guys are the best K clones a guy could ask for. Thanks for being a vital part of my life and for teaching me what it means to be a father. I love you!

To Rhonda & Charla: You two made this book possible by buying me the invaluable time to actually *write* and *promote* it! Without you? This would have been much, much harder. Thank you both so much! We love you!

To My Fellow Word People: Kayren Cathcart (PaperPolisher.com), Lanisa Fitzgerald, Kacie Dalton and my wife Kim (pulling double-duty). You ladies are the best! And you'll note I took your advice and removed the "make whooshing sounds to simulate blood flow." (See? I do listen!) Love you all!

To Ira-Rebeca: Thank you so much for providing the initial graphic design for Baby Codes. Your skill, insight and advice helped shape both the cover and course of this book in more ways than I can count. Thanks so much!

To Karen Hamilton Silvestri: Thank you for not only helping me whip my book proposal into shape, but for astutely pointing out that "101 Ways To Help Your Baby Sleep" is a subtitle, and not an appropriate working title. Let it be said here and now: if it weren't for your wisdom and advice, this would have ended up a much different book. Thank you!

To Lynn Jacobs: Best. Lifecoach. *Ever*. Thank you for helping me wade through the genesis of **Mills Creative Minds** and learn to trust in God's timing over my own. Your perfectly-timed nuggets of wisdom and grace hit home, every single time. Thank you!

To Keri Wyatt Kent & Jennifer Kennedy Dean: Your insights and encouragement in the areas of prayer, parenting & persistence helped shape me into the man and father I am today. I cannot thank you both enough for your books and ministries!

To MOPS International: Thank you, ladies, for letting me stretch myself as a speaker and, coincidentally, as a person. I hope my message of faith, hope and quiet obedience will resonate with you as you allow God to lead you to your next best step.

To my Mills Creative Minds Investors: Thank you for joining me on this sudden (and somewhat unexpected) turn of events. Your prayers and belief in me and my vision give me the strength I desperately need when my own strength fails. So grateful for you guys!

To God: Lastly (but certainly not least), I have to thank You, Father. Lord, this book started with You from Day One. Everything I've done up to this point and will do in the future is for Your glory alone. May you use me and any proceeds from this book as You see fit, Lord, for I will forever trust in Your divine timing, abundant providence and unconditional love. Thank You For Everything.

FOREWARD

BABY CODES
ANNIVERSARY EDITION

I have to admit, when I first started writing **Baby Codes**, I didn't think about the future. I didn't think this was going to be Book 1 of 5 (*it isn't*) or that I'd be featured on local radio and television stations (*I was*). I wasn't thinking about product tie-ins or partnerships or sponsors or *any* of that stuff.

Nope. All I was focused on was the need for parents to be able to get their kids to sleep. So *they* could get more sleep! That was it. More sleep for them, more sleep for you.

Now it's been ten years since **Baby Codes** was first published, and I figured it was time to give it some spit and polish. I went over the entire text with a fine-toothed baby comb, caught more than a few formatting errors and plumped up the whole thing here and there. Even now, I'm still pretty proud of how this book turned out, and I hope it gives you many years of additional slumber!

I used to spray some of the paperback copies of **Baby Codes** with a baby powder scented perfume, to give the reader an extra sensory experience. I'm not able to do that here (especially with the digital copies), but just know that if I could? I would. :)

Thank you for making **Baby Codes** a part of your sleep routine! I hope and pray your entire family gets the sleep they deserve!

Kevin Mills

INTRODUCTION

According to research by *Pregnancy and Birth* magazine,
today's newborns take an average of 56 minutes to fall asleep
at night. Parents typically have to get up two or three times to
calm them back to sleep. The "Average Mother"? She gets an
average of only three and a half hours of sleep a night. *A night.*
(Sound familiar?)

Sleep deprivation is not only annoying; it also creates
serious consequences. Sleepy parents are more ill-tempered,
forgetful and depressed. A severe lack of sleep also
contributes to reduced immunity levels and lower resistance
to infections, common colds, and the flu. (And I'm not even
going to mention the medical stuff like raised cholesterol,
high blood pressure, or increased levels of stress hormones in
general.)

The problem? You need a way to get your baby to sleep
soundly and consistently. (So *you* can sleep soundly and
consistently.)

The solution? It's in your hands.

Below are the **Top Five Reasons Baby Codes Will Rock Your World**:

1. It's Affordable. (Almost all combinations are absolutely free or easily affordable.)

2. It's Easy. (Each entry is short, to-the-point, and easy to remember.)

3. It's Organized. (**Baby Codes** is arranged by the five senses, so you can easily find the method that best suits you and your baby.)

4. It's Comprehensive. (I've read just about every baby sleep book ever published — so you don't have to. This book incorporates the most unique and effective solutions that simply work.)

5. It's *Guaranteed*. (Really. If you finish reading **Baby Codes** and you honestly and truly feel that *absolutely none* of the solutions inside helped you or your baby get more sleep, I will gladly refund your purchase price. *No questions asked.* Simply send the book along with your receipt to: **Baby Codes Refund, c/o Kevin Mills, Box 486, Como, CO 80432**.

How to Use This Book: Combinations Are Key

As you read through **Baby Codes**, you'll undoubtedly discover many of the ideas are blatantly contradictory. This isn't by mistake. In fact, there are two very good reasons for this: **1)** As you know, there is a wide assortment of baby sleep books written by other experts. And guess what? Some of them actually disagree with each other on ways to help baby get to sleep. **2)** Each child is unique. What works beautifully for one baby won't necessarily work for another. By the same token, what's discouraged or frowned upon for one might end up being *just* what *your* baby needs to sleep soundly at night.

So read this book with an open mind. *Stay flexible.* No

single approach will work with all babies all the time (*or even all the time for the same baby*). If one code doesn't do the trick, move on to the next . Combine two or three at a time, maybe switch up the order. You're free and encouraged to explore and experiment until you discover the right combination for unlocking your baby's sound sleep. (So *you* can finally get *yours*.)

You know that deep, restful sleep you've been dreaming of? Get ready. It's about to become a reality.

Legal Disclaimer: You should know that I am not a doctor. Or a pediatrician. Or a professionally trained baby expert by any definition. The ideas presented in Baby Codes are not intended to replace the sound medical advice you may receive from your preferred physician. (I am not that physician.) I am, however, a father with three sometimes adorable clones of my own, so I get it. I've been there. I know exactly how you feel: tired, exhausted, and desperate for some help. **I wrote Baby Codes for you**, *to provide you with 101 ways you and your baby can get the rest you need.*

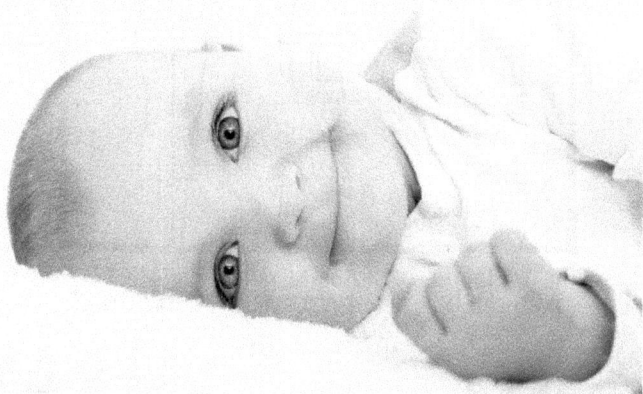

TASTE

IF YOU DIDN'T ALREADY KNOW, babies tend to explore their world by shoving as much of it in their mouths as quickly as possible. Sure, they prefer sweet stuff like breast milk or formula, but that's not going to stop them from grabbing anything and everything they can get their mitts on and giving it a formal taste test.

Thankfully, there are plenty of things you can introduce them to that are not only safe to suck on, but will actually bring you closer to your goal of Total World Domination.

(Or at least a sound night of uninterrupted sleep.)

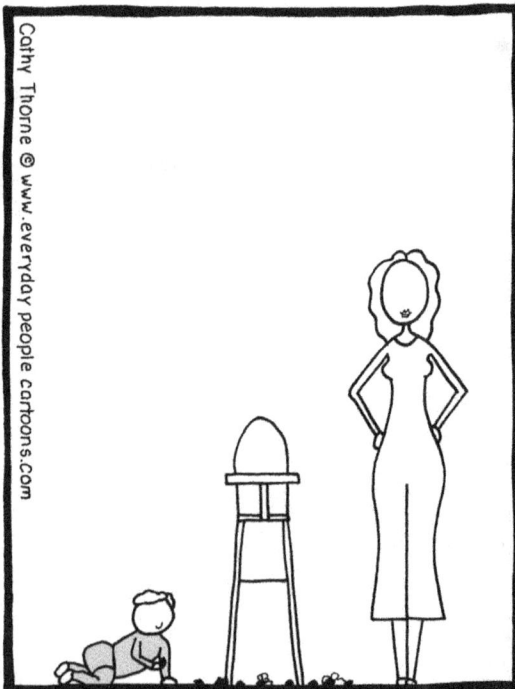

ACTUALLY, THE CRUMBS ARE INTENTIONALLY LEFT ON THE FLOOR TO DEVELOP FINE MOTOR SKILLS.

1. SAY HELLO TO HIS LITTLE THUMB

You might be opposed to the idea of allowing your child to suck on anything to speed up their sleep. Perhaps you even marched in a *No Pacifier* protest one weekend when you had nothing better to do. You may feel strongly about your stance (and be well-justified, no less), but guess what? If your little guy finds his thumb one night and grows deeply attached, there's really not a lot you can do about it.

Aside from sitting back and enjoying the silence as he sleeps in peace, that is.

The benefit of a baby sucking on his thumb versus a pacifier is obvious: it's permanently attached. No more searching frantically in a diaper bag while he's screaming in the carseat behind you. No more waiting for the dishwasher to finish the rinse cycle while he's bawling down the hall. No more midnight treks across the house to find and replace that misplaced pacifier that fell out of the crib.

Instead you'll hear nothing but the sweet, sweet sound of peaceful, thumb-sucking silence. See? Maybe thumb-sucking isn't such a bad idea after all, huh? (Of course, when he turns five and his thumb is his best friend, you might think differently....)

2. WATER: IT DOES A BABY GOOD

Water makes life so much easier, not to mention possible. A good **60%** of the human body is water. Our lungs are nearly **90%** water, and our brains are composed of a shocking **70%** water. Approximately **83%** of our blood is water, which helps us digest our food, transport waste and maintain proper body temperature.

Let there be no doubt: water is pretty important to our daily living. Thankfully, **breast milk is composed of 88% water.** This means if you're breastfeeding, your baby's *already* getting the majority of what she needs on a regular basis.

If she's over 6 months old, however, it might be time to supplement her with a few extra ounces of water a day. You should limit it to one or two ounces at a time, ideally administered after meals. This is especially helpful for babies with colic. Doctors typically advise that as long as the water isn't replacing a meal or breast milk/formula, giving your baby a few sips of regular ol' water a day won't cause any harm.

3. Break out the Bottle

Here's an interesting fact you might not know: bottle-fed babies actually wake up less often during the night. Why is that? Simple: formula typically takes longer for them to digest and contains more protein than natural breast milk. The more energy your baby has to expend in digestion means more crib time. And more crib time = **more you time**.

But let's be honest: it really just translates to more time for you to catch up on your sleep. (*You know you need it.*) So grab your bookmark and a bottle and get to it. I'll be here when you wake up. Promise.

Note: If your baby is breastfed, you may consider mixing your breast milk with some formula in the evenings. It may be just the concoction your baby needs to sleep those extra hours into the morning.

4. Find the Perfect Pacifier

There are a ton of different pacifiers out there. They come in a variety of colors, textures, shapes, and sizes — you'd think they were the latest Apple product, the way they're so aggressively promoted to parents.

So take note of this priceless nugget of advice: buy a variety of them.

Your kid is unique. As much as her or she might look like your clone (or their sibling's spitting image), they're going to have different preferences when it comes to ... well ... just about *everything*. And when it comes to something as powerful and vital as a pacifier, you really don't want to mess around.

Make a determined decision to dramatically increase your chances for binky success. **Buy a wide variety.** Short, skinny, thick, contoured. Try them all and try them often to see which one can claim the title of **The Ultimate Binky**.

Note: Want to stack the odds in your favor? Dip your preferred pacifier in a dab of jam or jelly before handing it off. That extra yum might be all it takes for your baby to establish a permanent bond with your binky of choice.

5. THE OMNIPRESENT PACIFIER

If you have a baby who's become dependent on a pacifier, you know what a godsend it can be. It's hard to imagine any other combination of plastic and rubber having such a powerful effect on a baby's state of mind. **Binky firmly in place?** All is well with the world. **Binky gone?** It ain't gonna be pretty.

Losing a pacifier in the middle of the night is even more traumatic for a baby. He wakes up knowing *something's* wrong, but he can't place his finger on it (literally), so he does the one thing he can do: he lets the world know about it. Thankfully, the solution to this problem is both simple and economical: *multiples*.

Rather than putting him to sleep with a single binky at

night, why not spread the love with *multiple* binkies? Instead of screaming for his BFF, all he has to do is reach around and voila! Reunited at last!

Note: If your baby's too awake to spread them around when you first lay him down, consider sneaking in and doing it when he's fully asleep. (You're going to need the practice as Santa, the Easter Bunny, and the Tooth Fairy anyway....)

Extra Note: *While you're busy expanding your pacifier collection, you might want to double-up on your Silky or blanket stock as well. When it comes to Binkies or Silkies? It truly is better to be safe than sorry.*

6. STOP STIMULATING THAT KID!

No, I'm not talking a back-to-back marathon of cartoons. I mean the chemical stimulants we often overlook as parents. You know, the ones found in food?

Fact is, there are a *ton* of stimulants in the food we eat. We don't notice it half the time because of our adult-sized bodies, but pump those same ingredients into our pint-sized clones? They'll become poster children for **Red Bull**.

Caffeine, of course, is the kicker (in so many ways). In addition to hiding in plain sight in our soft drinks, iced tea, and *Excedrin*, it's also sneaking around in chocolate and even in some kids' pain relievers. (I kid you not.) Stimulants sometimes masquerade under the names pseudoephedrine or diphenhydramine, so take a close look at that medicine bottle before letting Junior slurp down a spoonful.

Note: Not sure if a product's stimulating or not? Give 'em a taste-test during the daytime. In 20 minutes you'll know if it's got a secret pick-me-up inside it.

Oh, yes... you'll know....

. . .

7. Food Allergies Are Icky

They say anywhere from 3 to 7% of children and adults suffer from food allergies or some form of food intolerance. Funny thing about food allergies, though, is that they tend to be underdiagnosed by physicians and overdiagnosed by those affected. (As in, there's a little hypochondriac living inside all of us. Which, if you're a *true* hypochondriac, you're now freaking out at the image I just implanted in your head.)

While there's a wide variety of symptoms that could be caused by food allergies, the four common areas that are targeted are as follows: the respiratory passages, skin, intestines and brain. So if you think something's going on in one of those areas, you might consider checking in with your pediatrician ASAP. Or a professional allergist, if you're serious. (Or just seriously hypochondriac, if the shoe fits.)

8. Gripe Water: It's a Good Thing

When someone first told me about gripe water, I'll admit I was skeptical. An all-inclusive, homeopathic cure-all? Sounded too good to be true, if not downright scary. But after trying it out on my son's upset stomach and seeing the immediate relief and results, I can now honestly testify: *gripe water just WORKS.*

Gripe water is touted as a "homeopathic colic remedy" and helps in calming symptoms associated with baby colic and baby gas. It also relieves hiccups, stomach cramps, and teething discomfort.

So you may be wondering what, exactly, is in it? Basically, ginger and fennel and other natural goodness. Will it work for you? Who knows? But it's affordable, and what have you got to lose by trying it out? (Honestly, you can always give it away to other desperate parents if you don't find it to be effective. You know, make a new friend?)

9. Teething Tholuthions, Part 1

Have you ever wondered just how to know if your kid's teething? Start by looking for these possible signs: irritability, drooling, coughing, chin rash, biting or gnawing, cheek rubbing, ear pulling, diarrhea, low-grade fever, insomnia, or cold-like symptoms. (If you think that sounds an awful lot like PMS, you're not too far off.)

So what can you do to relieve her pain? Hand her a frozen washcloth.

Wet a corner of a washcloth, stick it in the freezer, and in thirty minutes you'll have the relief she needs. The frosty fabric will feel awfully good in her mouth while the icy cold will help numb her sore gums.

The best part? **It's absolutely free**, so you don't have to buy anything to try it out. (Unless you don't have a washcloth on hand ... in which case there might be more pressing issues to contend with ... such as basic hygiene....)

10. Teething Tholuthions, Part 2

Teething tabs look a lot like miniature marshmallows. They come in a dinky bottle too, so it's easy to glance at them and shake your head in doubtful skepticism.

This, of course, would be a serious mistake. Because within those teeny buds lies the power to stop a baby's teething woes flat.

The soft, homeopathic tablets dissolve instantly, they taste good, and there are no side effects. Best of all? *They just work.*

. . .

11. Teething Tholuthions, Part 3

Chilled rubber teething rings are a baby's best friend when they're teething. They come in a variety of textures and colors, and they're affordable.

Their magic lies in their ability to provide the counter-pressure that helps relieve achy teeth that are poking through tender gums. Combine that with the numbness that comes from the cold and your baby's pain will soon be a thing of the past.

12. Teething Tholuthions, Part 4

"Teething relief is a dish best served cold." - *Kevin Mills, Baby Sleep Specialist Guy*

As anyone who's had a mouthful of ice cream before bedtime knows, cold food can be a powerful gum number. Chilled applesauce, yogurt, or puréed peaches may be just what your baby needs to get through this trying time. Plus, they're a lot more nutritious than using a chilled washcloth or teething ring, which has zero nutrition whatsoever. (Or calories, if you're into counting.)

Other food suggestions include frozen bananas, frozen blueberries, chilled celery sticks, and, finally, frozen green onion stalks (not the actual white onion part). Although I haven't personally tried that last one, supposedly the juices inside the stalks are a natural pain reliever when they soak into the gums. Go figure.

13. Teething Tholuthions, Part 5

Legal Disclaimer: Before giving your child any drugs, always check with your doctor first.

There. Now that *that's* out of the way, let's get to relieving your baby's teething pain using the **Wonders of Modern Medicine.**

Giving your baby some Infant Tylenol with an Orajel chaser could be just what your baby needs to get her through her teething spell. Apply the Tylenol (or Baby Motrin) first, then immediately follow it up with a small smattering of Orajel on the offending area. By the time the Orajel wears off, the Tylenol begins to kick in. (It's like a swift, one-two punch against teething pain! *Biff! Bam!*)

Note: If Orajel doesn't seem to do the trick, many parents swear by Hurricaine Topical Anesthetic Gel. It provides some powerful numbing action and comes in flavors (Wild Cherry, Pina Colada, Watermelon, and Fresh Mint)!

14. Teething Tholuthions, Part 6

Okay, I really wasn't planning to write *six different entries* regarding teething, but two things happened: I kept running across good ideas, and my son conveniently had a nasty bout with teething as I was writing this section. So my brain was kind of on overdrive as I searched for solutions. (I figure it's better to provide you with *too many* options to choose from than *too few*, right?)

Because the pain in teething is coming from the teeth pushing up, some pediatricians suggest rubbing along the gums with your finger to provide some counter-pressure to help a baby feel better.

Consider putting a dab of Infant Tylenol (or Motrin, or Hurricaine) on your finger first, to allow for faster absorption. You might also want to slip one of those infant toothbrushes on first, for two good reasons: 1) To protect yourself from an unexpected bite-down crunch and 2) To provide your baby some extra massaging relief with the rubber bristles.

15. Cold Milk (It's What's for Dinner)

Hey, here's a fun physiological tidbit for you! Did you know that anything we eat has to be warmed up internally to our body temperature for us to digest it? It's true!

When you drink something cold, the tissues in your mouth, throat, and stomach are instantly cooled off. It then takes extra energy to heat those tissues back up to the appropriate body temperature.

What does this mean for your baby? Simply this: giving them cold milk will, essentially, **burn more calories** as their body heats it up inside. And burning calories makes babies sleepy. Very, very sleepy.

Note: This combination should only be used if your baby is over a year old, because giving milk (other than the breast variety) to a baby under that age could result in a pretty upset stomach. And that won't help you or your baby get any extra sleep.

16. Warm Milk (It's Also for Dinner)

Wouldn't you know it? Just as there's an argument for giving your baby cold milk, there's an opposite view regarding warm milk! So here are a few reasons you might want to warm that bottle up first.

Milk has tryptophan, that wonder ingredient that makes everyone super sleepy (commonly found in turkey, which helps explain the annual Thanksgiving comas across America every November). Warm milk raises your body's internal temperature a few degrees, which in turn triggers a "slowdown" response in our bodies. (Further perpetuating the stereotype of older people retiring to warmer climates when they slow down in life.)

Note: Again, only give your child <u>milk</u> milk if he's over a year old so his delicate tummy is developed enough to handle digesting the good stuff.

TOUCH

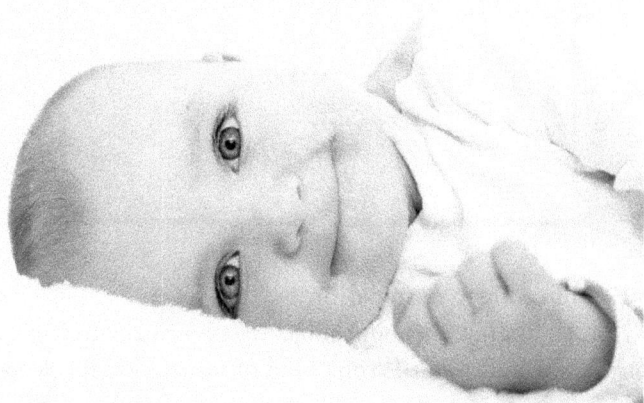

TOUCH IS one of the most well-developed of the five senses, especially in infants. Touching and being touched establishes a vital bond between a parent and her baby. Studies suggest the sense of touch contributes to a baby's cognitive and immunological development and increases overall attentiveness to the world around them. If you feel your baby is especially responsive to touch, the following **Baby Codes** will give you a head start on finding out how to use this unique sense to your advantage.

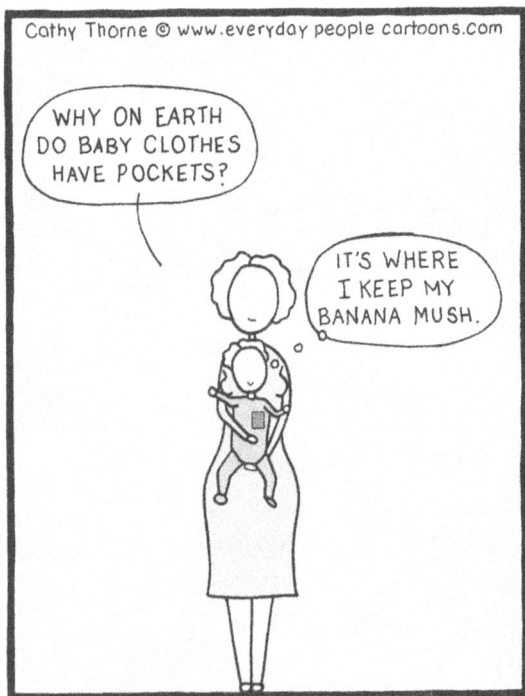

17. Find a Sleep Association

No, I'm not talking about subjecting your baby to endless observation at a clinic. (Wrong kind of association.) A sleep association is what each of us identifies as the final thing we remember before nodding off. So if the final image your baby remembers is being in your arms, sucking on a bottle or nuzzling with a blanket, there's a pretty good chance he's going to need that very same thing to get back to sleep when he wakes up in the dead of night.

Thankfully, you can help foster sleep associations and there's a wide variety of choices for you to offer your baby. My advice? Make it easy on yourself and choose something that's simple enough to recreate later. A soft blanky, a stuffed animal (*check for choking hazards*), a pacifier—something that's small and can easily fit in a diaper bag, purse or pocket.

Whatever you choose, however, **buy it in bulk.** Because you will lose or forget them in time. And trust me — you do *not* want to be without your baby's preferred sleep association token when it comes to bedtime.

You really, *really* don't.

18. Spoil Her with an Effleurage Massage

Infant massage has long been praised for greatly reducing tension, fussiness and irritability in babies, as well as aiding in their digestion. Effleurage in particular is supposed to have a positive effect on skin circulation, resulting in a relaxed, soothing (and sleepy) state.

Using only the lightest, most superficial touch, slowly glide your fingers over your baby's soft skin. For best results, start at the head and work your way down to the toes. Five short minutes of this and chances are good you'll *both* be ready to hunker down for the night.

Note: If your baby can't stop snickering or giggling while you do this, then effleurage is most likely not for him. Quickly move on to one of the other techniques and call it a night. Stop tickling that kid!

. . .

19. Give That Baby a (Sun) Bath!

Sunbathing. The nutrient-rich bath that time forgot.
Despite the bad rap the sun gets these days, moderate exposure to the sun has a lot of amazing benefits. Sunlight stimulates our happiness hormones (*endorphins*), inducing a sense of relaxation and wellbeing. It also helps our bodies generate essential vitamins such as Vitamin D to combat various illnesses. (*and over 16 different types of cancer!*)

So tomorrow morning, strip that baby down nekkid, find the softest blanket in the house, and let her soak up the sun in front of a window for a few minutes. (This is especially good to practice in winter time, when babies are typically bundled up like Chinese dumplings and rarely get any quality sunshine time.)

20. The Sweet Stretch

Everybody likes a good stretch. It releases tension and improves flexibility, and these things, in turn, help us sleep better. Stretching is even better when you've got someone willing to stretch your body *for* you, so you can fully relax and enjoy the full pull of it all.

The method is surprisingly simple. Holding your baby's opposing hand and foot, gently stretch her out diagonally an inch or two. Let her return back to her standard pose, allowing a few seconds to rest. Repeat. Switch sides to stretch out the opposite extremities once or twice, and you're done.

Ta-daahhh! Freshly stretched baby, ready for bed!

21. Booties to the Rescue!

"Hey! Who turned down the heat? It's freezing in here!"

Is this really what you want your baby to be thinking? Of course not. So perhaps you forgot that most babies — especially newborns — have trouble regulating body temperature? It's okay. There's a lot to learn about babies. Plus, we tend to forget what we're told in the hospital anyway, what with the childbirth process and a brand spankin' new baby handed over to us.

While newborns can heat their bodies efficiently, they have trouble *conserving* that heat (something about having no hair or shoes or anything…). So make it easy on 'em: slip on some soft socks or booties and let them bask in a new world of warmth and comfort.

22. MAKE YOUR OWN BABY BURRITO (AKA SWADDLING 101)

Trust me. When the nurses finally return your baby to you at the hospital, your first impression is going to be "burrito." It's okay; we all do it. Even those who don't crave Taco Bell on a regular basis. Your husband most likely thought something like "Lizard Burrito" when he looked down, but was sensitive enough to *not* blurt it out. I hope.

Simply put, swaddling is recreating the **Womb Paradise** your baby knew and loved by snugly wrapping her in a blanket. In addition to providing extra warmth and security, this also keeps her from being freaked out by her own jerking or startle reflex.

Most importantly? **It helps to calm your baby.** And a calm baby is a happy baby. And happy babies sleep more deeply.

23. SLIP HIM INTO A SLEEP SACK

An easy alternative to swaddling, **sleep sacks** are essentially spiffy sleeping bags designed just for babies. It just happens to have sleeves and a neckline to close it up, rather than a blasted zipper that always gets stuck when you go camping in some remote canyon overnight to impress your father-in-law.

But I digress.

At any rate, a sleep sack provides the same amount of cushy softness and comfort that swaddling does, *without* the smothering constriction. Now, while some babies love that feeling, others clearly don't. So it's up to you to closely observe them and then determine what works for your little one.

This method works best if you start when they're newborns and stay consistent. Trying to reintroduce it to a 9-month-old baby probably isn't going to have the effect you hope for.

Official **HALO SleepSacks** can be found here: https://www.halosleep.com

24. DASTARDLY DIAPERS, PART 1

Diapers are kind of a necessary evil when it comes to babies. You have to have 'em, but how do you know which ones are the best for *your* child? Cloth? Disposable? And which brand is ideal for your baby?

Again, this is going to come down to some research and experimentation on your part. First step? **Ask every parent you see.** I don't know if you've experienced this, but parents pretty much *love* to give advice on raising children, and we can be counted on to be very opinionated (and equally loyal) to whatever product solves our problems. So ask around and get some informed feedback on which diaper you should start with.

Second step: let the experiments begin! I'd suggest trying each one for at least a week to see if it's doing everything you hoped it would. Chances are good your box of diapers will last longer than that, but at least a week will give you enough time to decide what *works* and what *doesn't*.

And lemme just tell you — in my experience? — there are some diaper "solutions" which have been anything but. Bottom line? You'll want a diaper that's going to hold a night's worth of concentrated pee without bursting at the seams.

25. Circle the Ear and Repeat

This method worked wonders for me and my twin brother as a child. There we were in church, bored out of our minds and squirmy worms, but when Mom laid us down in her lap and gently circled our ears with her fingers? *Instant bliss.* All protests and fidgeting stopped immediately. We were utterly and completely incapacitated, transfixed and rendered powerless to the call of slumber suddenly whispering to us.

Note: In my experience? Circling behind the ear from top to bottom works best. Try the other direction and it's kinda like rubbing a cat backwards. It makes the cat crabby and your fingers get all icky. Avoid crabby ickiness by starting your circling out right, right from the get-go.

26. Dastardly Diapers, Part 2

Even if you've found the ideal diapers, there's still going to come a time when your baby develops a rash. And that rash is likely to affect his ability to sleep at night. So here's what you need to do:

• **Change diapers frequently.** Rashes form primarily because the skin is wet for too long. Keep a dry diaper on your baby *at all times*, checking it every hour if your baby is already developing a rash. (Be willing to change it at least once in the night as well. Or ask a loved one to… hint, hint…)

• **Avoid diaper wipes.** These can burn and actually increase the irritation. Consider using moist cloths instead. Yes, it's a hassle, but if your baby sleeps through the night? It'll be well worth it. Another option is to let the baby soak in a lukewarm bath between diaper changes, which helps clean the area more effectively.

• **Let 'em roam free.** That's right. If the problem is wet skin leading to a diaper rash, one solution is keeping the area as dry as possible… and that means no diaper *whatsoever*. (I know, you're shuddering at the idea ... I am too....)

27. SAY NO TO HOKEY POKEY

If you haven't experienced it already, there's going to come a time when you're doing everything you can to get your baby to stop crying and you're absolutely clueless to what the problem is. Thankfully, it could be a simple poking problem.

If there's an errant tag or piece of plastic or whatever stuck in your baby's sleeper or diaper, it's going to poke and irritate her. A lot. And the only way she's going to be able to tell you is with the God-given set of lungs she had when she first arrived on planet Earth.

So strip her down to nothing and start anew. You could spend your time inspecting her current diaper and sleeper for foreign objects, but why waste the time? Just grab a fresh set of everything* and begin again. Sleeper, diaper, the whole bit.

If she calms down right away, then you'll know there's a good chance she had a poking problem. And if not? Well ... you still have a good 100 other **Baby Codes** at your disposal.

Don't forget to grab a new pacifier, just to be safe.

. . .

28. Use Dad's Bare Chest

Babies constantly crave and need physical touch. Some experts would argue that it's just as important as getting enough food and oxygen. Touching your baby's skin is an excellent way to bond with them, *especially* when you're putting them to sleep.

So let your baby sleep naked on Dad's bare chest. If it's drafty, feel free to drape a light blanket over her, but remember that his own body heat will come into play.

Not only will this introduce direct, skin-to-skin contact, but it will allow him to better familiarize himself with his baby's unique scent and vice versa. (Gentlemen, don't make this harder than it is. If you're stanky and you know it, raise your hand. And take a shower. Please.)

29. Use Mom's Bare Chest

All the bonding benefits of lying on Dad's chest, only ... better. (I was going to say "enhanced," but that could easily be misinterpreted.... so I'm just going to leave that right there..)

30. One Good Stroke

Touch is one of the most important elements of a baby's growth because it's through physical contact that babies feel loved, protected and cared for. In addition to a gentle baby massage, another way to help your baby fall asleep is through the use of soft, stroking motions.

Starting from the juncture where the nose and eyebrows meet, slowly spread your fingers outward, gliding over the eyebrows to the edge of the temples. Wrinkled brows are a common sign of stress, so the more you can iron them out, smoothing the forehead into a relaxed, flattened state, the better your baby will relax.

Note: If you want to create a lasting illusion of contact even after you're gone, try moistening your fingers first. This will help press down and mold the eyebrows even more, helping them retain their newly chilled, stress-free state. Trust me, it works.

31. RUB HIS BACK THE RIGHT WAY

My second son was absolutely crazy about this idea. Immediately after he finished his bottle, I would lay him down in the crib (*complete with his favorite pacifier and Silky, of course*) and slowly start rubbing his back in a gentle, counter-clockwise motion. I'd do this for about 30 seconds to a minute and then give him a soft double-pat, tell him goodnight, and walk out of the room.

Granted, he typically sat up after I gave him those final pats and watched me leave the room, but then he would quickly flop back down and go right to sleep. Seriously.

Note: Consider alternating both the direction and duration that you rub until you find the perfect combination your baby likes best.

32. BACK TO STROKING

With your baby held against your chest overlooking your shoulder, use your free hand to slowly trace the contours of her spine. Start at the bottom and work your way up to the base of the neck, making sure to maintain constant contact (*otherwise it'll feel like she's getting poked in the spine, and no one really enjoys a spinal tap*).

The benefit to this technique is subtle. Because it's not a common place of contact, it typically takes a baby by surprise.

Suddenly, all their focus is on *that one sensation*, and when we focus intently on something, we tend to hold our breath. And holding our breath leads to reduced oxygen, and that, my dear friends, makes us feel super sleepy.

Now, if your baby convulses in a hysterical fit of giggling while you try this, you may want to abandon this approach and search for something a little less stimulating.

33. QUARTERBACK THAT KID

This is bound to be a favorite for those sports fanatics out there. After you've spent some considerable time with your baby, growing accustomed to their weight, speed, etc., try changing their bedtime routine by changing your grip.

Laying them sideways across your arm, face your baby away from you (*head resting on your palm, legs dangling by the elbow*) while keeping them nestled close to your hip or stomach. Many parents who have tried this method report it's especially effective with colicky babies or those with upset stomachs.

You might even find a football-themed sleeper out there to make the picture complete. Although I'd stop short of running around the house or barking "Hut One! Hut Two!"

Seriously. You've gotta draw the line somewhere, people.

34. SWITCHING FOR THE SANDBAG

You remember watching Harrison Ford as Indiana Jones in *Raiders of the Lost Ark*? The opening scene where he ever-so-carefully switches out a bag of sand for the sacred idol? Well, that nifty trick will work for you, too.

After rubbing your baby's back or chest for a few minutes, pause and let your hand rest lightly on top of him. Then resume rubbing again, pausing again 30 seconds later. The third or fourth go around, however, use your free hand to switch out your rubbing hand for a nearby stuffed animal.

Just like Indy, you'll want something with a similar weight and circumference as your hand. Too light, and your baby will know something's up. Too heavy, and your baby might very well cough something up. Like his liquid dinner.

So next time you're browsing the aisles for stuffed animals, keep this method in the forefront of your mind. And heed the advice given to Indy by that ancient knight guy in *Indiana Jones and the Last Crusade*:

"Choose wisely."

35. WARMER WIPES = SOUNDER SLEEP

Hey! Who wants to wake up in the middle of the night and have someone slap a frigid, wet washcloth on your butt? No takers? Then it's safe to assume your baby's not going to be too thrilled with the idea, either.

A good wipe warmer will not only heat the wipes from the top down (assuring a warm wipe every time) but will also have a built-in night light for changing. This is imperative when making sure your sleep-deprived wiping aim is as accurate as possible. Changing a morning diaper only to realize you missed a spot in the night isn't going to be fun. (Or fragrant.)

SIGHT

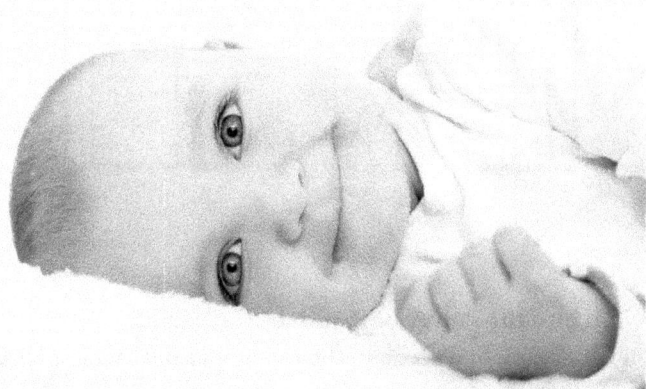

One of the first things a baby learns to recognize is her mother's face. Gazing at her mother as she's being nursed creates a strong bond where a baby feels both safe and secure. As her sense of sight develops, she tends to recognize more objects and sights around her that further enhance her sense of security. The sight-centric combinations in this next section will help her (and you) get some much-needed shut-eye.

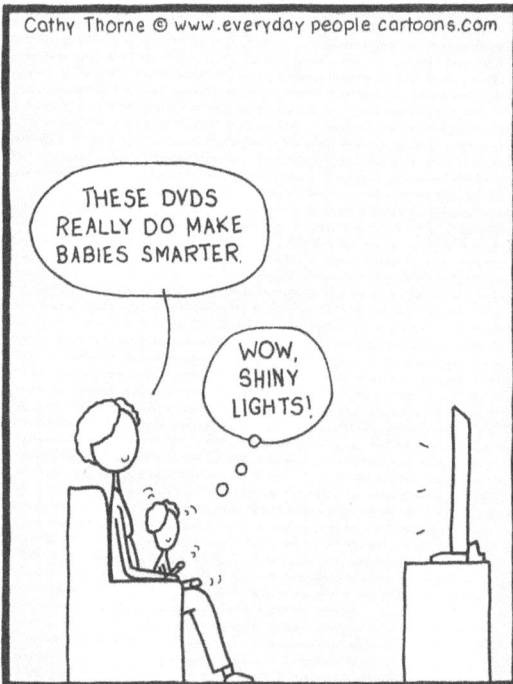

36. Tap into the Power of Bamboo

There's a pivotal scene in the movie *Kill Bill**, where Uma

Thurman's character faces off against Lucy Liu. They're in the garden, preparing to face off, and there's a bamboo fountain in the background, water slowly filling and emptying from it, wood gently knocking against wood (just before the fine ladies start screaming and slicing and dicing with their samurai swords).

Well, after some research I discovered it has a name: it's called a "deer chaser fountain." It's revered for simulating the calming sounds of a running stream, combined with the gentle rocking motion of the knocking bamboo.

Tranquil. Mesmerizing. *Sleep-inducing.* Everything your baby needs to sleep tonight.

Note: If you have absolutely no idea what I'm talking about, ask your husband or a macho male friend about the movie. They'll be glad to fill you in.

37. INTRODUCE HER TO THE DARK SIDE

A dark bedroom is pretty much a necessity for sound sleeping. So take a long look at your baby's room and decide what you're willing to do to reduce the amount of any outside light seeping in at any given moment.

Consider installing opaque shades to block out the bedtime and morning light that could intrude. This change alone could very well buy you an extra hour of sleep if you find your baby is one of those cocky little roosters who suddenly awakens when the first ray of sunlight hits the room.

38. DIM THOSE LIGHTS TO GET 'EM IN THE MOOD

Have you ever tried to go to sleep with four 75 watt bulbs lighting up your room like a Christmas Pageant? It ain't easy. But turning them off and depending on a dinky nightlight tucked away in a corner can sometimes be a recipe for disaster as well (*and scraped knees, and stepping on dropped toys, etc.*). My advice? Go for the middle ground: install a dimmer switch.

A dimmer switch does wonders in setting a room's mood for sleepy time. Crank it down before the bath; then when you follow up with the relaxing baby massage, you're ahead of the game. Turn on a little relaxing massage music at low volume, and whatever bedtime resistance your baby might have had will soon evaporate like a fine mist.

Sounds like a lot of work? It is. But then, you should probably ask yourself, "Exactly how badly do I want to sleep tonight?"

Uh-huh. Maybe it's worth it to call your handyman brother-in-law and get that thing installed. *Tonight.*

39. Soothed by the Flickering Flames

If you think your baby's destined to be a nature lover or avid camper, then this is the sleep solution you've both been dreaming of.

Pop in one of those virtual fireplace DVDs on your TV and let your child relax in the ambient beauty of the flickering flames. Many of these DVDs come stocked with multiple locales, ranging from a typical home fireplace to outdoor campfires or even a beach bonfire. As an added bonus, your baby may also be lulled to sleep by the comforting sounds of the crackling wood, chirping crickets or ocean waves crashing on the shore.

No wood to haul. No messy ashes to clean up. No smell of smoke. And the best part? It can play all night long. **All. Night. Long.**

Sweet dreams, Happy Campers. *Sweet dreams.*

. . .

40. One of These Things Is Not like the Other

One of the most common causes of nighttime wakey time for a lot of babies is misplacing their pacifier. He might slip away to la-la land with it safely between his lips, but hours of rolling around like a turnip tends to dislodge his teething treasure. Next thing you know, the redcoats are coming and he's appointed himself as the town crier while searching frantically for his long-lost friend.

Make it easy on the little guy by **creating a stark contrast** between his binky and his surroundings. Using a light-colored binky? Stick to dark sheets so when he wakes up he can easily spot it and pop it back where it belongs. (Invert the scenario if you want to go with the dark binky, lighter sheet motif.)

The less in-crib camouflage you create, the better. Baby awakes. Binky found. Disaster averted. *Quite possibly before Mom or Dad was even aware one existed.*

41. The Power of Moving Pictures

Please note: I am *not* talking about movies. Movies, for the most part, are a bad idea when it comes to putting your baby to sleep. Movies with characters and dialogue and sing-along-songs are designed to entertain, stimulate and generally keep an audience wide awake.

No, I'm referring to those backlit, photorealistic pictures that you typically find at a fantastical Asian buffet. Most likely it depicts a majestic mountain range or a cascading waterfall or a forest canopy. As you stare at it, you quickly realize you're utterly mesmerized. Why? Because a subtle element of it (water, clouds, etc.) is actually *moving*.

Hang one on the wall across the room from the crib and your child will *also* be absolutely mesmerized. Plus, it doubles as a night-light. (Bonus!) Combine this idea with a soothing nature sounds CD and you have yourself a surefire recipe for wooziness.

42. OUT OF SIGHT, OUT OF MIND

I'll be honest. This is one of my absolute favorite bedtime techniques. I didn't read about it anywhere in the other baby sleep books I devoured, but simply dreamed it up when I first became a full-time, Stay-at-Home Dad. It worked for me, and I'm betting it will work for you, too.

Can we all agree that the initial goal of bedtime is the closing of the eyes Ideally, we all hope and pray that sleep will soon follow, but in the beginning? **It's all about the eyes.** Or the *eyelids*, to be specific.

With your baby flat on her back in the crib, slowly back away as you simultaneously lower yourself down. If she's at the age where she watches your every move, she's going to be staring you down in sheer fascination and confusion. (And let's be honest, she has good reason...)

But here's the kicker: as you lower yourself out of her line of sight, her eyes continue to rotate downward, thus simulating the heavy, drowsy sense that precludes sleep. I know, it sounds absolutely ludicrous, but I assure you — **it works wonders**. Once is usually sufficient, but feel free to repeat as often as necessary. (You'll know if it's necessary...)

43. GET READY, KIDS! IT'S FAMILY SLIDESHOW TIME!

See? Your eyes are *already* glazing over at the mere thought of sitting through an evening of watching your parents' slideshow of their latest international trip.* Now imagine exposing your baby to a random stream of your unorganized digital snapshots, and you'll soon see the hidden potential of this **Baby Code**.

To be even more effective, you could make nighttime-specific slideshows by using darkened photos, pictures of their bedroom at night, etc., to help reinforce the idea that nighttime is quiet time. Avoid the bright, action-packed outdoor montages of last week's picnic; such photos will *not* help your cause. (Another option is to create a family-specific slideshow, focusing on the faces you want your child to be most familiar with as they grow up.)

So where do you begin? If you're a Mac user, **Apple** makes it easy with their phenomenal **Photo** app (*which comes pre-installed on every Mac you buy*). But don't worry; there are plenty of free photo editors for you PC users out there as well. My suggestion? Stick with Google's excellent **Picasa** software (http://picasa.google.com). It'll be more than enough to get you through the night.

*Note to my parents: I am not, in any way, referring to your vacation slideshows. Which are always riveting, informative, and extremely exciting. Extremely.

44. SHOW HIM THE LIGHT OF DAY

I should point out that this isn't the same as direct sunbathing. In addition to allowing limited time in direct sunlight, there's reason to believe that even exposing your child to *indirect* light in general will help him sleep better.

A study from **John Moores University** reported that babies who were exposed to twice as much light during the day (*typically between noon and 4 p.m.*) became better sleepers at night.

The theory is that higher light levels encourage the development of their biological clocks and circadian rhythms. This, in turn, regulates various bodily functions, such as the secretion of melatonin. And melatonin is a key player when it comes to sleep and establishing healthy sleeping routines.

So slide up your shades, pull those curtains aside, and open up those windows during the day. Flood your house with the sleep-inducing goodness of natural light! Your baby with thank you. (*And your spouse, and yourself, and anyone else sleeping in the house at night.*)

45. HYPNOTIZE AND VISUALIZE WITH iTUNES

When you think about it, there's really only a small handful of fantastic, life-changing inventions when it comes to babies. Baby wipe dispensers, **Boppys**, **Bumbos**, and everything in between. But when it comes to technology? There's simply no question: **iTunes is about to become your bestest friend ever!**

This one's a double whammy. Why? Because in addition to distracting your child with music, you also have the added benefit of a wide variety of visually mesmerizing, hypnotic animations to choose from. What's more, you can download custom visualizations to plug directly into **iTunes**, so you can experiment and discover which one is best suited to lull a fussy baby to sleep. (My recommendations? Search online for the plug-ins **Punkt**, **Fizz**, **Fountain Music**, and **Snow**.)

The best part? **iTunes is absolutely free.** You can download it for both Mac and PC by visiting www.apple.com/itunes. Once installed, just open **iTunes** and start playing a song. Then go up to **View** in the menu, scroll down to **Visualizer**, pick a favorite, and you're set.

Let the mesmerization begin!

.   .   .

46. Begin Operation Blackout

The inspiration for this idea came from my in-laws. When I first met them, they were proud owners of a pair of cockatiels. Pretty birds ("pretty birds"), but *holy cow* are those things loud! I pity anyone who's foolishly standing beside their cage when they release an earsplitting shriek. Put a cover on their cage at night, however, and you'd hardly know they were there. *Kind of like pet rocks.*

While putting a thick blanket over your baby's crib would not be a wise choice (please don't do that), there *are* ways to create a simple and effective sensory deprivation canopy that will do the job. If you're not a crafty handyperson, find someone who is and explain what you're wanting. Give 'em some PVC pipe, some black, breathable fabric, and a few hours to spare. Chances are he'll be able to whip up a decent cover for that kid that will keep her visually isolated throughout the night.

Note: Again, make sure the fabric is both lightweight and breathable. You want it to block out light, not oxygen or airflow. Also keep in mind that if your black canopy is supported by stark white PVC pipe or wood, you're going to need to invest in some decent spray paint to help it blend in a bit.

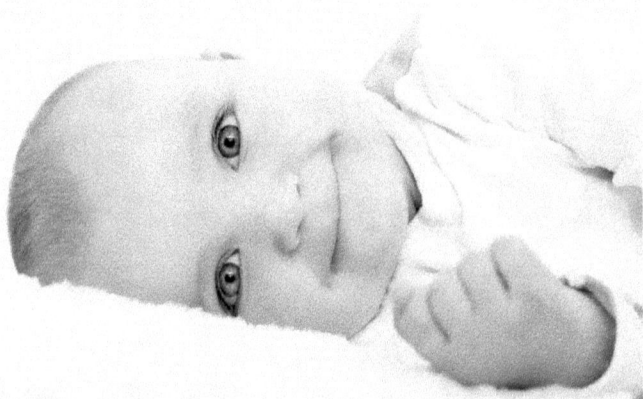

SMELL

ALTHOUGH TOUCH IS CONSIDERED the most well-developed sense, smell is *by far* the most advanced of the five. In fact, experts insist that babies develop their sense of smell *while still in the womb*. After birth, babies use this sense to quickly make associations with their parents, creating a sense of safety while in close proximity to them. Capitalizing on the strength of your baby's sense of smell will help you find the exact scent-infused **Baby Code** that will help her sleep.

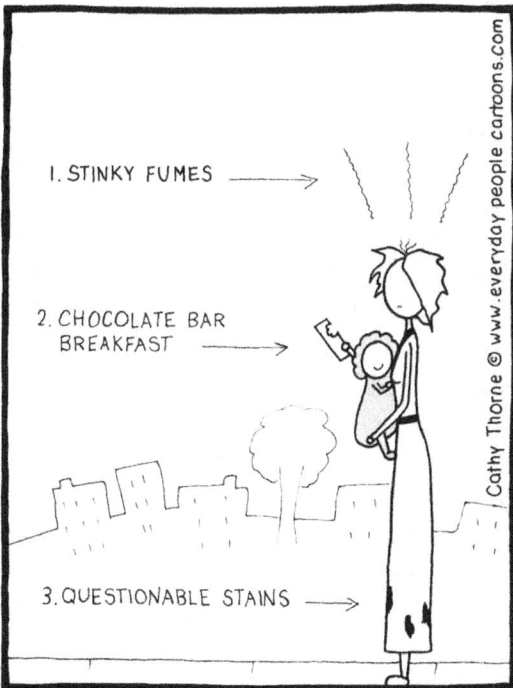

I USED TO CROSS THINGS OFF MY "TO DO" LIST, NOW I CROSS THINGS OFF MY "I'D NEVER DO" LIST.

47. Bath Time: The Aromatic Appetizer

Giving your baby a bath shortly before bedtime has a ton of benefits. It's a nice, leisurely ritual that serves as a nightly cue, communicating "It's almost time for bed." It helps to shift your child's body temperature, slowing them down as their inner core heats up, making them ready to conk out. Finally, a bath is considerably easier and less dangerous than holding them up in the shower or hosing them down in a sink.

One way to enhance bath time is with some aromatic baby bubbles. While there's a wide variety to choose from, the most popular is probably **Johnson & Johnson's® Bedtime® Bath** with **Lavender & Chamomile**. In fact, J&J attests that using their product, followed by a short massage and quiet time, is *"clinically proven to help babies fall asleep easier and sleep through the night better."*

Wow. Who can say no to *that*, huh? I mean, once you use the phrase *"clinically proven,"* it's pretty much a done deal. We're sold. For best results, however, you should probably invest the time necessary to determine exactly *which* scent your baby responds to best and then run with it.

48. Nipple Juice (It's Powerful, Powerful Stuff)

So an infant's sense of smell begins in the womb, long before he sees the light of day, right? What's more, your baby can find Mom's nipple by its scent less than an hour after birth! How's *that* for amazing?

This **Baby Code** taps into the comforting Mommy mojo that is your breast milk. Sprinkle or spray some of it onto the blanket before you lay it down with her. Sure, you might think it's nasty, but your baby? She'll love it. In fact, she'll be comforted by sweet-smelling, sleep-inducing scent of heaven.

Note: Moderation is the key here. Don't dowse the thing. Just a short spray or a few drops will do the trick for a good week. (At which point you should wash it and start over again. Please.)

49. Scent Switching 101

This is almost as sneaky as my earlier **Touch Baby Code #34**, *Switching for the Sandbag.*

Whether you realize it or not, your baby's attached to your distinct scent. All that time you were cuddling with him and hugging on him and squeezing him and calling him George? He was huffing in the naturally fragrant goodness that is **you**. And this is a good thing.

Why? Because at the end of the week, you now possess a powerful tool in your Sleepy Time arsenal: **your scent-saturated shirt or nightgown.** Spread it out flat beneath the crib sheets and your powerful, unique aroma will continue to lull them to sleep all night long. Sounds bizarre, but *it works*!

50. Spread Your Scent Around

Okay, so maybe the idea of handing over a sweaty T-shirt to your baby just isn't sitting well with you. You've tried the deep breathing exercises and called your counselor and close friends, but the obsessive-compulsive side of you is kind of sort of screaming in protest at the very notion.

Not to worry. There's a solution for you too. Instead of using the natural muskiness of your dirty laundry, use the next-best thing: your unique fragrance of choice.

Spray a small misting of *your* preferred perfume on her blanket or crib sheets (during the day when she's not on them, of course). That's it. Your job here is done. You've now transformed the crib into a heavenly-scented, Mother-like haven. Smells like Mom!

Note: For best results, try to be consistent. Stick to one or two scents to allow your baby enough opportunities to associate you with the smell. And for the love of Pete, do not accidentally choose something with pheromones in it! That's just craziness in a bottle.)

51. STANKY BLANKY GOODNESS

As a compliment to the stanky shirt/nightgown suggestion ("Scent Switching 101"), you might also want to keep a blanket on hand during bedtime.

Placing it between you and baby while you rock her for a few minutes, it'll quickly absorb your scent and infuse it deep into the fabric. Then when you lay her down in the crib, simply place the blanket down alongside her. Mom might disappear, but at least your baby will still have a fragrant memento to comfort her throughout the night.

It's sneaky. It's stinky. It works.

52. VANILLA SOOTHES BABY SOULS

You're not going to believe this.

A few years ago there was a study at **Gettysburg College** where a group of babies were exposed to a vanilla scent before and after a doctor's visit. The findings? *They were remarkably calmer* when compared to the group of kids who weren't. It's true!

Of all the scents out there, **vanilla is one of the most effective when it comes to reducing anxiety and nervousness.** So when you're thinking of how you want the baby's room (or crib, or bath…) to smell, consider choosing plain ol' vanilla. Not only will it help soothe your baby, but there's a good chance it'll help calm *your* nerves as well.

. . .

53. A Scent-ual Massage

We've already established that giving your baby a massage helps them calm down before bedtime. Well, one way to enhance the effectiveness of that time is by adding some natural, stress-relieving scents into the mix.

Mixing two drops of aromatherapy oil with 4–6 fl. oz. of baby oil is more than sufficient to do the job. (It's powerful stuff. Please resist the temptation to overdo it.)

Some recommended oils (the most "gentle" ones) are **Chamomile, Lavender, Rose, Neroli, Sandalwood, Tangerine,** and, of course, **Vanilla**.

54. Please Clear the Area, Part 1

Especially in the early months, your baby is going to need clear canals in order to breathe. Eventually, they learn to alternatively breathe through their mouth if their nasal passages are blocked, but in the beginning? **The nose knows best.**

Clearing the nose is best accomplished with one of those rubber bulb syringe things. In addition to this, you might want to add some saline drops to help moisten and loosen up the mucus before you try to suction it out. (Chances are, it's gonna be wet enough.) While you can always buy saline drops at your pharmacy, you can just as easily make them at home by dissolving 1/4 teaspoon of salt in 8 ounces of warm water.

Then it's just a matter of swabbing 'em up and sucking 'em out. *Go slow...* nobody really likes getting something shoved up their nose, no matter how much they'll appreciate it later. (*Doesn't that sound like such a parent thing to say? "You'll thank me later." Only this time it's true. We hope....*)

55. Please Clear the Area, Part 2

So you swabbed and sucked that sucker, but it's still not enough? Then perhaps it's time to use the steaming power of ... steam.

Shower steam, to be precise.

Go to your bathroom with your baby, shut the door, and turn the shower on full blast, as hot as it'll get. Then take a seat beside it while the shower does its thing. In mere minutes you'll be surrounded by gloriously sticky steam and all the nasal-blasting power that's contained within. (Note: You should *not* step into the shower with your baby. That would be a definite no-no. It's only purpose here is to generate the steam. Nothing more.)

An alternative option is using a cool mist vaporizer in the bedroom. While some will allow you to add a menthol solution to help clear the air, I wouldn't recommend this if your child is less than 2 years old. (*Always read the directions or ask your pediatrician if you have doubts.*)

56. PLEASE CLEAR THE AREA, PART 3

Bedroom inhalant allergies typically result in stuffy noses and midnight waking spells. Thus, you'll want to make sure your baby's room is as dust-free as possible. This means removing any fuzzy blankets, down comforters, or other dust-collecting magnets (fuzzy toys, etc.).

If you think your baby is particularly allergy-prone, a quality HEPA-type air filter might also provide some relief. (Plus, the white noise it generates could even help baby fall — and stay — asleep.)

SOUND

KEVIN MILLS

JUST LIKE WITH their ability to smell, babies develop their sense of hearing long before their actual birth. While in the womb, a baby can hear a wide variety of sounds ranging from a mother's heartbeat, sudden loud noises, or even music. They can also differentiate between the sound of a mother's voice and that of a stranger. Sounds play a key role in a baby's language learning as they develop. Tapping into your baby's sense and appreciation of sound will allow you to find the perfect code or combination that will soothe them to sleep.

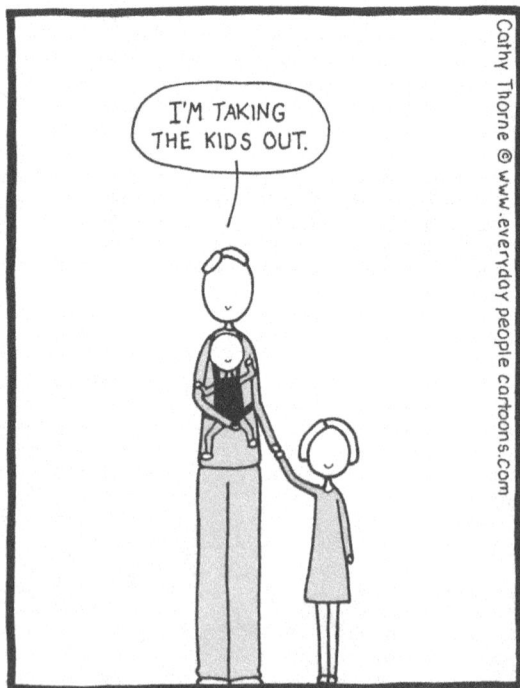

I'M TAKING THE KIDS OUT.

Cathy Thorne @ www.everyday people cartoons.com

THE SEXIEST MAN ALIVE!

42

57. Post-Rock 'Em to Sleep

If you've never heard of **Post-Rock music**, you're about to become the proud owner of a very happy, very sleepy baby. Post-Rock is composed of instrumental music created with typical rock instruments, but relying on downbeat tempos and lush, sweeping melodies. Critics often dismiss it as simplistic, predictable and repetitive — which is *exactly* why your baby will love it.

There are a handful of talented Post-Rock artists out there, but I'm going to narrow it down to my top picks, just to make it easy for you: **Hammock, The American Dollar, Lowercase Noises**, and **Lights & Motion (Christoffer Franzen)**. Don't waste another moment. Go to **iTunes, Amazon** or wherever great music is sold and grab one of their albums today.

Lowercase Noises — *Marshall, Vivian, Blake, Seafront, Ambient Songs*

Hammock — *Maybe They Will Sing for Us Tomorrow, Mysterium, Universalis, Silencia, Oblivion Songs*

The American Dollar — *Ambient One, Ambient Two, A Memory Stream, The Technicolor Sleep*

Lights & Motion / Christoffer Franzen — *Bloom, Phenomenon, Wide Awake, While We Dream,*

58. The Art of Noise

It might seem like a no-brainer, but it's worth mentioning that babies will sleep deeper and for longer amounts of time if they're in a quiet environment. **Noisy places make for**

cranky babies. And cranky babies make for sleep-deprived parents. So take note.

In addition to ensuring baby gets the cue that quiet times are rest times, you may also want to help them make the connection by actually *introducing* noise into their daytimes. I know, that sounds contradictory, but stay with me, here.

Say your baby's awake? Time to crank up the stereo a bit, turn on the TV, or do whatever you're comfortable with to add to the aural onslaught. It doesn't have to be loud, but some background music that the two of you can enjoy and dance to? That's good stuff.

59. WHITE NOISE ROCKS!

White noise is described as *"sound that contains every frequency within the range of human hearing in equal amounts."* So, what does white noise mean to you? Peace and quiet, my friend.

Peace. And. Quiet.

In layman's terms, the steady stream of monotonous white noise acts as a filter against *external noises*, effectively masking the distractions outside the room and helping your baby calm down quickly.

Thankfully, there is a wide variety of white noise CDs and digital downloads to choose from. Google "baby white noise" and you're sure to find the right white noise solution for your baby tonight.

60. SING-A-LONG WITH IPOD & FRIENDS

This is super easy, completely free, and chances are good you already have the three things you need to get started: **1)** a baby who needs sleep, **2)** an MP3 player, and **3)** a voice.

Before picking up your baby, grab your media play of choice and select a playlist that you're comfortable singing along to. It doesn't necessarily have to be stuffed with America's Top Lullabies or anything, but you might want to avoid heavy metal, punk, or country for the time being. (*Actually, you might want to avoid country songs altogether... depending on your location and tolerance level...*)

Playlist selected? Volume comfortable? Earbuds in place? You're clear for takeoff!

You may now pick up your child and entrance them with your soft, soothing singing.

"*But I can't sing!*" you protest? Not to worry — your baby doesn't *know* this. What's more, he's not going to be judging you like a scornful **American Idol** judge or anything. He's just thrilled to have you singing to him. Really! Trust me (and trust yourself). It's a **Baby Code** worth trying at least once.

61. The Call of Nature, Baby

The sounds of nature typically produce a peaceful and calm ambiance for the listener, allowing the mind to disengage from the day's active pace.

There's a wide range of natural sounds to choose from: waves on the beach, a gentle rainstorm, distant thunderstorm, jungle rainforest, crackling fire, running water... the list goes on. Chances are pretty good your baby's going to quiet down to at least *one* of them.

As an alternative to buying a complete nature soundtrack, consider some of the more affordable options such as individual MP3s, nature sound websites (www.SoundSleeping.com), and what's freely available in your local library's music section.

. . .

62. OPEN UP AND SAY "YAWN"

We've all experienced it. You're stuck in a meeting or a classroom, desperately trying to fight off the pasta-induced coma from lunch when you look across the room and see one of your peers let out a tremendous, irresistible yawn. You try to fight it, but you can't. Seconds later? You're yawning in response, like some kind of twisted echo. Why is this?

Well… we're not really sure. Heck, we're not even sure why we yawn at *all*! Scientist big-wigs think we primarily yawn because our bodies are trying to fight off sleep and draw in more oxygen to the bloodstream, in an effort to help keep us awake. Funny thing, though… by the time we're yawning, it's usually too late. We're already circling the rim of unconsciousness and it's only a matter of time before we cuddle up with our pillow.

Thankfully, you can use this contagious nature of **The Yawn** to your advantage. When you're walking the baby around the room, settling into the nighttime routine and giving her all the necessary visual and auditory cues that it's time to go to bed, go ahead and fake a yawn or two. Chances are good she's going to mirror you and slip that much further down the rabbit hole of sweet, sweet dreams.

Fun Fact: Scientists also say that simply reading the word YAWN can often cause people to yawn as well. So... are you yawning yet? (Be honest. I know *I* am…)

63. TURN THE RADIO ON

In today's satellite and internet radio-centric world, the radio is an often forgotten resource. I readily admit it's been years since I've intentionally turned the radio on. I question why should I ever let someone else determine what I'm listening to? But maybe that's just me.

Nonetheless, the radio might be just what your baby needs to get to sleep. Here are two good options to choose from:

1) Tune it to talk radio. Hearing the endless drone of a chattering talk show host might be just the thing for your baby to mentally disengage. (It works for me....)

2) Tune it in to sheer static. Just like the white noise described in **Baby Codes #59**, the monotony of the radio static could help lull your baby into the deepest sleep he's had in days.

Either way, radios are cheap to come by, and the sound waves are completely free.

64. EXTREME SOUNDPROOFING 101

I have a friend who is extremely sound sensitive when it comes to sleeping. Even the slightest noise outside his house will wake him up and rob him of hours of rest and slumber. That is, until he came up with the perfect solution. He sound-proofed his bedroom with carpet.

On the walls.

Using his analytical, engineering mind, he reasoned that the most effective and economical buffer between the bed and outside noise was a good layer of carpet along the walls. The fibers absorb sound going in and out of the room, enveloping him in a sweet womb of silence throughout the night.

So there you have it. Think your baby is extra sensitive to nighttime noises? Consider adding a few layers of carpet or padding to your bedtime strategy. If your baby's room has sound-reflecting wood or tile floors, you may want to find an area rug to help quiet it down.

65. ASLEEP IN A HEARTBEAT

Up until the shocking trauma of being born into the world, your baby's entire existence was in the warm confines of a womb. It was there he was fed and cared for, completely secure and protected. And you know what sound he heard all day, every day? **Your heartbeat.**

The soft and rhythmic sound of your heartbeat served as a constant reminder of his safety and security, and that sound *still* holds the power to calm a fussy baby, immediately transporting him back to a place of peace and quiet.

Consider investing in one of the many high-quality heartbeat CDs that are available to you. Some have lullaby music or nature sounds as a backdrop, but your best bet might be the simple sound of a lone heartbeat.

66. WIND CHIME SLEEPY TIME

Different sounds have different effects on the body. A soft, babbling brook will have a vastly different effect on a person's well-being than the sound of glass breaking, nails on a chalkboard or screeching tires. Many parents believe sounds affect a baby in utero and regularly expose their unborn child to music or peaceful sounds while she's still forming in the womb.

There's a wide variety of natural and peaceful sounds to choose from, but one of the most popular is the wind chime. Whether it's made of bamboo, wood, glass, or metal, wind chimes are a fantastic way to instantly create a peaceful, meditative atmosphere for your child.

Whether you choose to go with a physical chime (accompanied by a soft fan) or digital (MP3s, CDs, etc.), you really can't go wrong. Experiment with different variations if you're keen on finding the exact chime your child responds to best.

· · ·

67. ANIMALS TO THE RESCUE!

If you find you travel with your baby a lot and don't always have a CD player around to play white noise or heartbeat sounds, you're in luck. **Sleep Sheep** is here to save the day!

This cute, cuddly creature does more than snuggle up with your loved one; it plays a variety of soft sounds to help your child calm down and drift off. Whether you want white noise, sounds of nature, or the reassuring sound of a heartbeat, the **Sleep Sheep** has you covered. Plus, they come in a wide variety of animals, including **Giraffe, Dolphin, Turtle, Lady-bug,** and **Polar Bear**. (Note: They have no plans to manufacture a **Sleep Scorpion** anytime soon, so don't bother asking.)

You can order the **Sleep Sheep** directly through the website (www.cloudb.com), or Google it and you'll find plenty of places that sell this lovable scamp.

68. FINDING NEMO AT NIGHT

Placing an aquarium in the bedroom can be extremely relaxing for a baby. Soft lights, dancing fish, and quiet purring of a motor as it churns out a constant stream of bubbles can all work wonders to induce sleep. Plus, they provide a constant and consistent sleep association. Every time the lights go down and she sees the aquarium, she'll remember it's sleepy time.

Two things to consider if you decide to install an aquarium in your child's room. First, make sure you pick one with lights that aren't glaringly bright. Bright light won't help your Princess hit the pillow. Be sure to ask around and do some research before you buy.

Second, you're gonna need to maintain that thing and clean it often. As fun as fish are to watch, they require a lot of fish food, and fish food makes fish poop, and pooping fish make for a stanky tank after too long.

To Summarize: **Yes** to aquariums. **No** to stanky tanks.

69. SAY A BEDTIME PRAYER

I believe prayer is, without question, the single most important thing you can do for you and your child. Not only in helping them get to sleep as young children but by guiding them throughout the rest of their lives as they grow from childhood into adulthood.

We love our children deeply. As loud and frustrating and crazy as they can be, the truth is we all really *do* love our kids. By praying for them nightly, we're effectively committing them back into the hands of the One who gave them to us in the first place. We're able to recognize them as the precious gifts they are and entrust their future into His loving hands, both immediately and eternally.

Don't know where to begin? Try this:

"Lord, thank you so much for my baby. Thank You for bringing him into my life and allowing me to show him love and care for him. Please help him sleep through the night and rest peacefully, and give me the strength and patience to give him what he needs as a young child. We love You, Lord, and we pray this in Jesus' name. Amen."

70. TALK 'EM DOWN

Your baby doesn't talk, but believe it or not he's soaking up far more of the world around him than you realize. He may not understand the specific words you're speaking to him, but he can easily sense the underlying tones and meanings.

As you're holding him in your arms, administering the final bottle of the night, talk to him about what's happening (*and going to happen*). Describe how sleepy he's feeling, how his eyelids are becoming very, very heavy and will be closing shortly, and how he'll soon be lying down in the crib and falling soundly asleep.

Why it works: whenever we focus our attention on something — reading a book, listening to someone speak, drawing a picture — we're unconsciously **holding our breath.** It's true. When we *really* focus, we're holding our breath. We can't help it. Fewer breaths = less oxygen. And less oxygen?

Well, that makes for a nice, drowsy bedtime.

71. CLEAR THE EARS

A common ailment that prevents babies from sleeping is the notorious ear infection. These tend to appear after a common cold or sinus infection, and there are specific symptoms to look for that might help you stop it before it gets worse.

- Cold symptoms (nasal drainage changes from clear to yellow or green)
- Sudden fussiness
- Sudden fever
- Pulls or tugs at ears
- Doesn't want to lie flat
- Diarrhea*
- Reduced appetite*

*The bug that often causes an ear infection also has an effect on the gastrointestinal tract.

*If you believe your child has an ear infection, it's always best to have him checked out by his pediatrician before things get out of hand.

. . .

72. Super Sleepy Story Time, Part 1

Babies begin to learn and understand language well before they're able to speak it. Talking to your baby on a regular basis plays an important role in their cognitive development. In addition to this, the more she hears your voice, the more comfortable and safe she'll feel in your presence. (Especially during times when she can't see you, like in the car.)

If you can read and hold your child at the same time, feel free. But if they're at an age where she'll grab the pages or you're just uncomfortable with the idea, feel free to sit in a comfortable chair beside her while she lies in their crib. (Another option is to place her in a **Bumbo** on the floor.)

What to read? Anything you'd like. Read a toddler favorite such as any of **Dr. Seuss's** classics or *Harold and the Purple Crayon* by **Crockett Johnson** (my older son's favorite). Or you can read aloud the novel you're reading these days. Or a short story. Or a magazine article. Cookbook. Munitions manual. Whatever floats your boat.

Truthfully, there isn't a *wrong* way to do this. Just read aloud in a quiet, soothing voice, and you're golden. Eventually, you might not even need to read aloud because your very presence in the room could be enough to calm your baby down for bedtime.

73. Super Sleepy Story Time, Part 2

If you're the creative type (or just plain desperate), you're going to love this combo.

After your baby is prepped and ready for bed, begin softly telling a story to him. You could talk about a classic fable, about your day (or the day you *wished* you had, if you want to rewrite it), about the future — whatever you want. Share a memory, make it up on the spot, it's completely up to you. You're in charge.

Storytelling can be an extra powerful sleep combination when you tell the *same* story every night, again and again. It's a unique way to bond with your baby, it establishes a quiet bedtime routine, and it's one of the most effective language-learning tools available. (And did I mention it's **free**?)

74. SUPER SLEEPY STORY TIME, PART 3

If you're too tired to read aloud and too left-brained to come up with your own spontaneous stories, don't fret. There's yet another option for your child to fall asleep to: **Audio CDs**.

Just visit your local library (either physically or online) and you'll find a wide variety of audio books for children. Whether your preferred medium is cassette tapes*, CDs, or MP3s, the library has everything you need. And it's free!

If they have stories that are geared for babies, fantastic. But don't worry if they don't. It's more important to play some kind of story to help your child sleep than it is to find "the perfect story." At this point, you just want to see if playing a story at night helps your baby settle down whatsoever, not expand their young minds through classical or modern literature.

A "cassette tape" is how music and books used to be consumed and shared back in the 70's and 80's, kids. You will need a "cassette tape player" to make them work. And most any garage sale you visit will have one. (Trust me ... they just will....)

TIME & SPACE

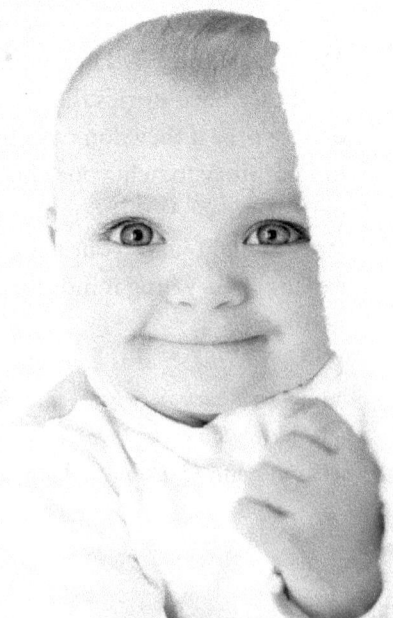

ASIDE FROM THE primary five senses, the two other ways babies interact with the world around them are through **Time** and **Space**. Granted, they're not as aware of these things or how they affect them. But *you* are. And that's a key point because with that awareness comes the power to affect not only what your baby experiences, but *when* and *where*. The ideas associated with **Time** and **Space** will be some of the most important **Baby Codes** you use (if not *the* most important ones).

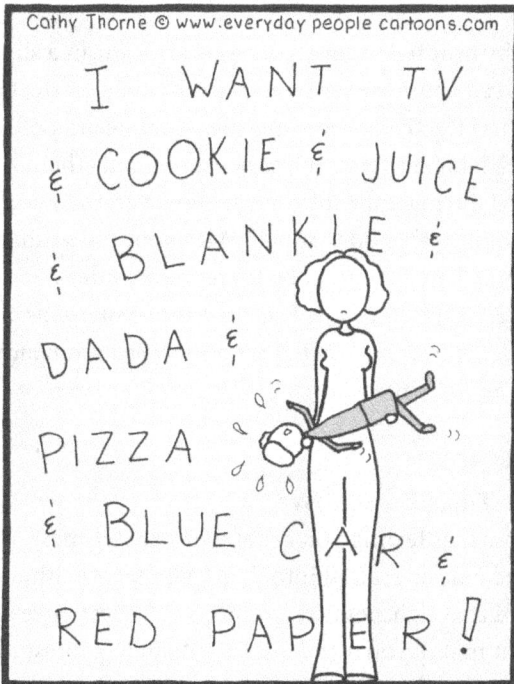

Cathy Thorne © www.everyday people cartoons.com

I WANT TV & COOKIE & JUICE & BLANKIE & DADA & PIZZA & BLUE CAR & RED PAPER!

WHEN THEY CAN'T DECIDE WHAT THEY WANT, THEY NEED A NAP.

75. Bounce, Baby, Bounce

You say your baby's not old enough to enjoy the benefits of bouncing? Not to worry. With a little effort and creativity on your part, she'll be reaping the rewards in no time!

The easiest (and least jarring) way to bounce with your baby is on a **Swiss exercise ball.** You've undoubtedly seen them while flipping through retro cable channels at night. Some super-skinny chick is bouncing on one, barking orders into a mic with a smile, all while barely breaking a sweat. Well, today *you're* the one on the ball, leading your exercise crew of two.

With baby **cradled securely** in your arms (or in a sling) and feet spaced apart for support, *gently* bounce on the ball. That's it. This effectively recreates the womb feeling of motion, which babies tend to like because it puts them at ease. If you jogged during your third term, however, then you'd better get comfortable on that ball. With your kid's inherited motion quota? You just might be there for a while....

*Note: Alternatives to a Swiss ball are a mini-trampoline or simply the edge of your bed. Whichever method you use, remember the keyword here is **gentle** bouncing. This isn't Jazzercise, you know.*

76. Change Their Perspective

You know that feeling you get at work sometimes? You're stuck behind a desk, stuffed into your cubicle or behind a counter, and that tightness creeps into your chest once again? The one that makes you just want to scream in protest of the sheer monotony of it all?

Believe it or not, babies need a change in environment too. So don't just carry them to bed in the same position, night after night. Mix it up. Try something new. Instead of cradling them in your arms, prop them up on your shoulder once in a while. Let 'em look around the room, enjoy a change of scenery, experience their little lives from a different perspective. Show them a closet, a new corner of the room, a window view.

Granted, their eyes might only register a shapeless blobs (depending on how old they are), but at least it'll be a *different* shapeless blob than the one they've grown accustomed to.

77. SWIVEL THOSE HIPS!

I'm going to venture a guess and say the chances are good that I'm the only one who's used this technique. However, because I can personally attest to the fact that it's worked consistently when it comes to putting my son down, I'm going to include it.

The gist of it is simple: standing up and cradling your baby in your arms (facing up), slowly swivel your hips in a repetitive motion.

That's right. **Just like a hula dancer.** Admit it, you've always wanted to try this but were too paranoid you'd get laughed at. Well, here's your chance, right in the dark privacy of your own home. Initially you may want to keep it simple with a clockwise direction. But if that's not doing the trick, I highly recommend the "Figure 8" swivel. (Just like it sounds ... draw a figure eight with your hips.)

Remember to keep it **slow**. You don't want you or your passenger becoming so dizzy that you have to lie down on the floor. (On the other hand, lying down to rest is kind of the whole point ... so ... ah ... follow your instincts.)

78. GO FOR AN OLDE TYME CARRIAGE RIDE

Just because you *can* buy a newfangled stroller for the

same price as a used car doesn't mean you *should*. Nor is it necessarily the best solution for knocking your beloved baby out. Why not ask Grammy if she still has that buggy thing in the cellar or attic? Those bouncy springs might be just what you need when it comes to wiggling and jiggling your baby off to dreamland.

Note: You may want to test the thing with a full-sized watermelon first. Just to be on the safe side. Because, you know, you can always buy another watermelon if it doesn't work out as you expected.

79. Naptime: Regularly Scheduled Programming

In case you don't know by now, babies need naps. And *lots of them*. On average, a newborn will need approximately **14 to 15 hours of sleep a day**. (I know, you're drooling at the idea. That's normal.) Naps are crucial to making sure they get the rest they need to grow into the happy toddlers of the future.

This sometimes means rearranging your schedule to adjust to your child's unique sleep preferences (at least during the first few months). If your baby is naturally a night owl or an early bird, see if there's a pattern and try to adjust to it. Over time you'll be able to nudge her to adjust to *your* preferred schedule for naps, but in the beginning? Don't fight **Mother Nature**.

Babies who have regular naps tend to be better-rested and happier for the remainder of their busy day. They will eat better, listen better and learn better. They'll likely have more positive energy and will be less cranky. They'll also sleep better at night.

Why? Because while their bodies and brains aren't utterly exhausted, they'll still be tired enough to fall asleep on cue at their regularly scheduled bedtime.

If you haven't already mapped out a naptime routine, take a few minutes to do so now. (You'll be glad you did. Really, really glad.)

80. NAPTIME: AFTERNOON DELIGHT? THINK AGAIN

Afternoon naps? Great idea. Late afternoon naps? Not so great.

As you determine the best naptime schedule for your baby, take extra care not to slot one too late in the afternoon. Too close to dinnertime, and you're going to have to face the sobering fact that your baby is fully rested and full of energy a few hours later.

Skipping the afternoon nap altogether has consequences as well. By doing so, they might be too exhausted to eat anything whatsoever, prompting you to put them straight to bed. Sure, they might sleep like rocks for a good chunk of time, but when their hunger pangs set in later they're not going to care whether or not it's light outside. They'll want what they want, and they'll want it *now*.

Try to plan your day well ahead of time so you won't become trapped in a late afternoon dilemma.

81. NAPTIME: SYNCHRONIZED SLEEPING

Some of you Type A, always on-the-go individuals are probably going to balk at this idea, but I'm including it anyway. It's for your own good. Trust me.

So sit down, take a deep breath, and read this suggestion with an open mind:

You need to sleep when your baby sleeps.

There. I said it. Let the vocal protests begin. But not until after you hear the reasons why. Whether you admit it or not, you're pretty sleep deprived. You're up at all hours of the night, you're stressed out and you're probably a bit cranky. At the same time, you're overwhelmed with guilt about the state of the house, the stacks of dirty dishes, and the mountain of a laundry pile that continues to grow. It's time to face the facts: **you're exhausted.**

Get some sleep! As soon as your baby is down and out, *you* need to lie down. For you to be the parent you want to be — the patient, loving, giving parent your baby needs — you can't keep overextending yourself. It just won't work.

Please. Give yourself a much-needed break and start making your sleep a priority today.

82. DAYTIME: CELEBRATE INDEPENDENCE!

As much as your baby depends on you every day, part of your responsibility as a parent will be to teach him to become more fully independent. One of the best ways to do this is to begin having select times during the day when you leave the room, allowing him to be by himself for a few minutes.

By experiencing regular alone times during the day, he'll eventually learn that it's actually *okay* for him to be by himself. His sense of security and independence will grow, and he'll be able to cope better when his social security blankets **Mommy** or **Daddy** aren't in plain sight.

The dividends of this come at night, when your newly independent baby discovers he's actually *okay* with being left alone at bedtime. (Or even better, when he wakes up in the dark dead of night.)

83. DAYTIME: DON'T STOP DRIVING

If you're lucky, you've got one of those babies who can

sleep anywhere, at any time. In a park, on the train, at the zoo, on a plane, in a box... with a fox. (You get the idea.) But some babies will only take naps in one place consistently: the car.

If that's your baby and he consistently knocks out while you're going to and fro, I only have one suggestion: don't stop driving.

Experts say that anything less than a 45-minute nap won't make a sufficient dent in your baby's sleep quota. As in, even if he nods off for a few minutes at a time, his body won't *feel* like he took a nap. This means you may very well end up with Mr. Cranky Pants if he wakes up too early.

Maybe he needs the vibration of the car, or maybe he'll be just as happy sitting in a parking lot while you read a book (or tilt the seat back and take a nap yourself). You'll have to see what works and what doesn't. But take heart: even if you idle the car for an hour it's probably still cheaper than hiring a babysitter these days.

84. DAYTIME: MAKE 'EM LAUGH

Kids are wired for fun. They're constantly curious, incessantly inquisitive, and the epitome of the word "uninhibited." Thus, they're typically ready to laugh at a moment's notice. Which is perfect, because the more you can make them laugh during the day, the better they're going to sleep at night.

Here's the skinny on why laughter will rock your socks off:

- It stimulates deep breathing
- It improves lung capacity and increases oxygen levels in the blood
- It instantly reduces the levels of stress hormones (epinephrine and cortisol)

- It increases brain endorphins and serotonin (natural mood enhancers)
- It improves the circulation of both the cardiovascular and lymphatic systems
- It boosts the immune system
- It encourages self-confidence, creativity, and social communication skills
- It promotes better sleep (Ta-daaah! Ladies and Gentlemen, we have a winner!)

So pull that clown costume out of your closet, grab your red nose, and slap on that rainbow wig. It's time to put on a show, people! The bigger they laugh, the harder they'll fall! (... *fast asleep, that is!*)

85. DAYTIME: SLOW DOWN, BABIES AT REST

On the other hand, maybe your baby doesn't like to be yanked about whatsoever. Maybe she craves the status quo. In this case, make a concerted effort to slow her world down by slowing yourself down. Run fewer errands, plan fewer events, visit fewer people and places, do fewer things.

There's a common problem that occurs for parents of newborns: they don't know how to slow down for their baby. Most likely you've been an active part of the workforce up until now, and the shock of having so little time and energy to do what seemed like a simple job (*in theory*) is confusing, confounding and frustrating to you.

Here's the thing: **you have a new job now.** You're not necessarily going to get the perks, the pats on the back or the encouraging feedback you're used to. Prepare for this. But also make a point to consciously downshift the frantic pace of your life.

Don't try to stuff everything into your day with a jam-packed schedule. If you're always coming home late from music lessons or baby activities, it's downright stressful... on both you *and* your kids. **Kids need downtime.** Lots of it. And they're depending on *you* to make sure they get it.

Just say No to busy, hectic parenting.

You'll be glad you did.

86. DAYTIME: A BABY IN MOTION TENDS TO STAY IN MOTION

...that is, until they fall fast asleep from exhaustion.

Rather than embracing the mellow side of life, you may find it more effective for you and your baby to seize the day with as much gusto and activity as possible. Numerous studies show that people who engage in vigorous exercise through the day tend to sleep better and more soundly at night.

A car ride, a stroller tour, a baby sling, an infant swing — find what works best and plug it into your routine. It should be noted that keeping your baby in motion is *especially* effective if your baby is colicky, because a lot of babies with colic can be soothed <u>only</u> by motion and movement.

87. DAYTIME: WALK OFF THE WILD SIDE

One of the best ways you can ensure your child sleeps soundly tonight is to take her for a leisurely stroll this afternoon. In fact, based on a study in **The Huffington Post** a few years ago, a 20-minute stroll can help hyperactive children calm down as effectively as Ritalin.

Why does it work so well? There's a handful of theories, but most conclude that the combination of fresh air, sounds of nature and perpetual movement has a subtle calming effect. Plus, the outdoors are filled with a wide variety of **engaging**

stimuli (*blowing wind, beaming sun, chirping birds*) that trigger our involuntary attention. This serves to refresh us for when we have to concentrate on something later.

If you find you and your baby are tired of being cooped up inside all the time, take this idea for a test-drive and see if both of you don't end up sleeping better because of it.

88. Daytime: The Word of the Day Is M-E-L-L-O-W

If you find your baby is extra clingy throughout the day, perhaps you'll consider indulging this side a bit more. The idea is to fill your baby's "Parent Time" tank so much that when bedtime arrives she'll be fat and happy with all the quality time you two shared.

A great way to do this is to stay as attached to your baby as possible through the day. Hold her, stroke her, kiss her, and just enjoy your time together doing everything or absolutely nothing. (For you Type A mothers out there, this could be good therapy for you as well.)

By fostering a mellow daytime filled to the brim with physical proximity, your baby may very well carry a lasting sense of peace and serenity into the night.

89. Bedtime: Self-Soothing 101

Ah, self-soothing. I ask you: is there any topic that's more emotionally charged when parents talk about putting their children to sleep? I doubt it. so here we go...

Side A insists it's cruel and inhumane, that ignoring a child's cries for help has a lasting and detrimental effect on their growth and well-being. Side B, on the other hand, argues that letting their baby cry it out was the *only* way they established a workable sleep routine.

So what exactly does self-soothing look like? Basically, it's putting the baby down to sleep and then allowing him to calm himself down, rather than intervening to calm him down directly. Just like crawling takes time for them to pick up, babies also have to be given time to learn how to self-soothe.

The primary benefit of having a baby who picks up this skill is they're independently able to calm themselves down when they awake in the middle of the night. (And let's face it — that's a pretty huge benefit.) This skill also translates well when they get older and are in other stressful situations, such as being dropped off at a nursery or daycare or staying with family (or whenever you're out of their sight, for that matter).

Some parents teach their babies all at once, checking on them infrequently to reassure them. Others start gradually, sitting next to the crib the first night and then moving farther and farther away on subsequent bedtimes. Eventually, you'll be able to tell the difference between cries that say "I'm hungry" or "I'm dirty" or "I'm just plain lonely." (You may consider reading *Secrets of The Baby Whisperer* by Tracy Hogg for more information on how to identify and translate your baby's cries.)

90. BEDTIME: CONSISTENCY IS *STILL* KING

In the same way consistency is a vital part of setting a naptime routine, it's even more important when it comes to bedtime. A consistent bedtime routine provides children with the cues they need to understand what time it is. (Remember, babies don't wear watches.)

It's important for you to do the *exact same things* at the *exact same times* before putting your baby to bed. There are all kinds of things you can choose from: singing a song, reading a book, taking a bath, etc. The routine elements themselves aren't nearly as important as keeping them quiet, low-key, and **consistent**.

91. BEDTIME: AVOID THE GRAND TOUR

If you're walking around the house during bedtime, darting from one end to the other as you get your baby ready for bed, chances are good you're going to be up longer than you anticipate.

When you start preparing your baby for bedtime, make an effort to move in **one direction** and one direction *only* — toward the bedroom. If you find yourself giving your baby a bath, then going to the kitchen to make a bottle, rebounding to the office to feed while you surf the web, and finally heading in the other direction off to bed... well... you're going to end up confusing and inadvertently stimulating that child.

Start to picture yourself as a Mommy Monorail. Baby gets onboard and away you go down the track. There's no turning left or right, and there's no turning back. You might make a stop once or twice (bath time, story time, etc.), but only move in one direction. Before you know it, you'll both be arriving at your final destination: The Land of Sweet, Sweet Dreams.

92. BEDTIME: START EARLY OR FINISH LATE

An important question you have to ask yourself is *when* you want your baby to go to sleep. By this, I mean when she's completely out, down for the count, and you're free to have some quality time. (And by "quality time" I mean "fall into bed in a heap." Not the *other* definition... *wink, wink...*)

A rookie parent's mistake is to severely underestimate how long the bedtime routine actually takes. You'd be surprised how fast time flies when you're filling it with bath time, story time, a final feeding, etc.

Your best bet? **Start the routine early.** Start the bath *early*. Get them in pajamas *early*. Break out the binky *early*. Get a head start on every single aspect of the routine so that if and when you run into setbacks along the way it won't disrupt the entire evening. You'll be ahead of the game.

Remember: the sooner *they* get to sleep, the sooner *you* get to sleep. (And that's the whole reason you started reading this book in the first place.)

93. Bedtime: Comfort Comes First (Yours, That Is...)

As you find yourself focusing intently on how to help your baby sleep, it's easy to forget about your own personal needs. Blinded by the endless stream of diapers, feeding, burping, napping, and just plain surviving, new parents are often shocked to realize how much they've neglected themselves.

Believe it or not, pulling off a successful bedtime routine starts with **you.** The parent. So take a moment to assess yourself before launching into the fray.

Kick off your shoes, let down your hair and take a deep breath. Put on some quiet music. Engage in some deep stretches. **Do whatever comes to mind that will make you feel relaxed, comfortable, and at peace.**

There. Feel that? That sense of calmness seeping through your veins? Now you're ready for whatever the night holds in store for you — sleepy baby or not. (Good luck. You got this.)

94. Bedtime: Location, Location, Location

As you select where to lay your baby down for the night, take special consideration when choosing a location. Your two

KEVIN MILLS

primary options? In her crib by herself or in bed with the parents.

Option number two (also called *co-sleeping*) has pros and cons. On the pro side, the familiarity and warmth of being close to mommy may help her feel more secure, thus helping her sleep better. You also won't have to tromp across the house for nighttime feedings because baby will be right by your side. Finally, some studies indicate that the regular breathing patterns of the parents help the baby regulate her breathing as well. Those are the upsides.

The downsides? Pretty serious. If you or your spouse are deep sleepers, there's a good chance one of you could accidentally roll over and suffocate the baby in your sleep. Not coincidentally, studies also show a higher rate of *Sudden Infant Death Syndrome* for babies who sleep in their parents' bed.

Either way, it's a personal decision that you and your spouse will want to talk over before committing to a course of action. Regardless of where you choose to end bedtime, remember that your baby will want to fall asleep in the same place every single time, so be prepared to help her along by building a consistent routine.

95. BEDTIME: KEEP A SUPER-SECRET SLEEP DIARY

Okay, it doesn't really have to be super-secret. But I'm a sucker for consonance, so I decided to sneak it in there. (*See what I'm saying?*)

By keeping a record of your child's sleep signals, you'll have a better idea of what to look for when you need to identify their sleep-readiness. This will better assist you in seeing the patterns so you can anticipate the ideal nap and bed times.

. . .

96. BEDTIME: THINK WARM THOUGHTS

Babies don't really care for being cold. (I know… crazy, isn't it?) They spent the first nine months of their lives developing in the balmy 98.7 degree paradise that was your womb. Then they were thrust into the world and the quest for thermal self-regulation began immediately. Thankfully, you're there to help.

It's especially important to keep your baby warm throughout the bedtime routine. Transitioning from a warm bath to a warm towel to your warm arms and finishing with a warm breast and a warm bed is a surefire way to keep your baby calm and relaxed.

Place a warm towel or a heating pad (set to low) on the sheets to warm them while you're getting him ready for bed. Test it with your hand and then remove the towel or heating pad just before laying him down for the night. Moving from the warmth of your body to the warmth of the sheets makes for an easy transition. Everybody wins!

Note: You might also use a hot water bottle or water-filled balloon if you're feeling adventurous. Or just plain lucky.

97. BEDTIME: QUALITY TIME WITH YOUR CLONE

Here's an idea: Instead of rushing through the bedtime routine in an effort to get your baby to sleep *as soon as humanly possible*, what if you slowed it down just a notch? After the bath, the bottle, and the blanketing your baby in bed, don't leave.

Pull up a chair. Whisper to her. Rub her back. Listen to some music. Check e-mail or play **Words with Friends** or **Candy Crush** or whatever's popular now on your phone. Text your spouse in the next room. Read a book. Pray.

For some babies, just having you there beside them is all it takes for them to feel secure enough to fall asleep. Your very presence provides them with the comfort they need.

98. BEDTIME: CHOOSE YOUR TIME WISELY

As much as I've mentioned rearranging your schedule to accommodate your baby's, there's another alternative to consider: adjusting your child's bedtime to suit your needs.

For instance, if you find that putting him to bed between 7 and 8 p.m. typically results in an early-morning, 6 a.m. wake up call, you might want to stretch it out a little bit longer at night. On the flip side of this argument, if you keep the baby up late for a 9 p.m. bedtime, then you're going to be sacrificing some serious quality time with your spouse (or your precious alone time to decompress from the day).

There are tradeoffs to either decision, so take the time necessary to decide what your priorities are. You'll be one step ahead of the game.

99. BEDTIME: PREPARE FOR CABIN DECOMPRESSION

There may be nights when you put your baby down for bed and they're just not tired. (I know. Shocking, isn't it?) So what's a parent to do?

Give them time. With or without you, that's your choice. But sometimes your child will just need a few extra minutes to settle down and unwind. Maybe you'll need to let them cry for a few minutes before they find a comfortable position and fall asleep. Perhaps they need some extra time to listen to you as you recount the day or talk about the future.

You'll need to make the final call on what you think your baby will need on nights like these. But if you have a plan ahead of time, you won't have to scramble for a solution when you find yourself here unexpectedly.

100. BEDTIME: YOU ARE NOW ENTERING THE NO-FUN ZONE

I'm a fun-loving person by nature. Making people laugh is my secret hobby, and it's even more rewarding when my kids are the ones with the chuckles. But at bedtime? That's when we put fun back in the box and settle down.

It's incredibly important that you make the last 30 minutes before starting your bedtime routine a time of rest and relaxation. It needs to be as peaceful as possible, stimulation-free.

No hide-and-seek. No tummy tickle time. No swinging the baby from her feet or throwing her into the air. None of it.

Set the nighttime tone. Dial it down. Get more sleep. (See how easy that was?)

101. BEDTIME: HIT THE SLEEPY STUPOR SWEET SPOT (OR "Don't Lose That Drowsy Feeling")

Try to put your little angel to bed too early or too late, and you're likely to find her halo has transformed into a pointy set of horns. They'll either be too wound up or too exhausted and cranky to tuck in for the night.

The key? Putting them to bed when they're *drowsy* but still awake. Look for the telltale signs: yawning, blank stares, rubbing their eyes, and general fussiness. Once you can identify the precursors to a drowsy baby, you'll have a short window of opportunity in which to put them to bed.

The result? Your baby starts to associate their bed with that drowsy feeling and, of course, the sense of falling to sleep. Problem solved.

· · ·

A Few Signs Your Child Is Getting Tired:

Newborns—yawning, frowning, clenched fists, blank stares, and, of course, uncontrolled crying.

Older Babies—eye rubbing, fretfulness, separation anxiety, and a sudden loss of interest in toys or playing. And crying.

Toddlers—slow to respond to questions, clumsy physical movements, emotionally tense. And (*any guesses here?*) crying.

CONCLUSION

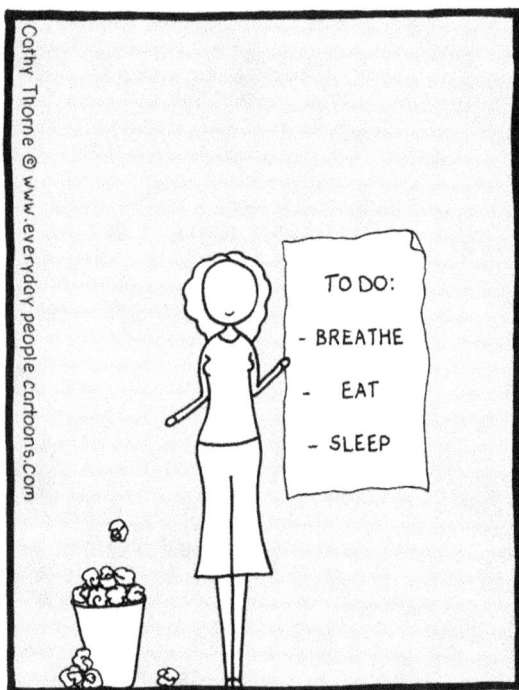

THERE'S ONLY ONE REAL "TO DO" LIST.

There you have it: 101 unique, powerful, and yes, sometimes bizarre ways you can help your baby get to sleep. **101 Baby Codes** to unlock the hidden safe of slumber that's locked away deep inside your Little Man or Princess. 101 ways that you can choose from to achieve the ultimate goal: your sound sleep!

By now you probably have a good idea which codes will work with your baby and which won't. Whether they responded to **Taste** or **Touch**, **Sight** or **Smell**, **Sound** or **Time and Space**, my hope and prayer is that you and your baby are on your way to being 100% happy, healthy and well-rested.

I want to personally thank you for purchasing **Baby**

Codes! My goal is to get this book into the hands of tired parents everywhere, so if you feel this book helped you in your bedtime success, please consider recommending it to someone you know who could use it.

Sweet dreams!

Kevin Mills

SUGGESTED READING

CUTHBERTSON, JOANNE
SCHEVILL, SUSIE
Helping Your Child Sleep Through The Night.
Main Street Books, February 1985

DOUGLAS, ANN
Sleep Solutions for Your Baby, Toddler and Preschooler: The
Ultimate No-Worry Approach for Each Age and Stage
(Mother of All Solutions).
Wiley, May 2006

EZZO, GARY
On Becoming Baby Wise: Giving Your Infant the Gift of
Nighttime Sleep.
Parent-Wise Solutions, Inc., September 2006

FERBER, RICHARD M.D.
Solve Your Child's Sleep Problems.
Simon & Schuster, January 1985

GIORDANO, SUZY
ABIDIN, LISA
Twelve Hours' Sleep by Twelve Weeks Old: A Step-by-Step
Plan for Baby Sleep Success.
Penguin Group USA, January 2006

GORDON, JAY
GOODAVAGE, MARIA
Good Nights: The Happy Parents' Guide to the Family Bed
(and a Peaceful Night's Sleep!).
St. Martin's Griffin, July 2002

KARP, HARVEY, MD.
The Happiest Baby on the Block: The New Way to Calm
Crying and Help Your Baby Sleep Longer.
New York: Bantam Doubleday Dell Publishers, 2002.

KIMES, JOANNE
LACCINOLE, KATHLEEN
YOUNG, LESLIE
Bedtime Sucks: What to Do When You and Your Baby Are
Cranky, Sleep-Deprived and Miserable.
Adams Media, November 2007

LAVIN, ARTHUR
GLASER, SUSAN
Baby & Toddler Sleep Solutions for Dummies.
For Dummies, September 2007

LAWLER, JENNIFER
The Complete Idiot's Guide to Sleep Training Your Child.
Alpha, October 2006

MACGREGOR, CYNTHIA
Getting Your Baby to Sleep: Lifesaving Techniques and Advice
So You Can Rest, Too (Mommy Rescue Guide).
Adams Media, June 2007

MINDELL, JODI
Sleeping Through the Night: How Infants, Toddlers and Their
Parents Can Get a Good Night's Sleep.
Harper Paperbacks, March 2005

MOORE, POLLY
The 90-Minute Baby Sleep Program: Follow Your Child's
Natural Sleep Rhythms for Better Nights and Naps.
Workman Publishing Company, January 2008

PANTLEY, ELIZABETH, AND
SEARS, WILLIAM, MD.
Perfect Parenting.
New York: McGraw-Hill / Contemporary Books, 1998.

PANTLEY, ELIZABETH.
The No- Cry Sleep Solution: Gentle Ways to Help Your Baby
Sleep Through the Night.
New York: McGraw-Hill / Contemporary Books, 2002.

SEARS, MARTHA
How To Get Your Baby To Sleep: America's Foremost Baby
and Childcare Experts Answer the Most Frequently Asked
Questions.
Little, Brown and Company, August 2001

SEARS, WILLIAM, MD, AND WHITE, MARY

SUGGESTED READING

Nighttime Parenting: How to Get Your Baby and Child to Sleep.
New York: Plume, 1999.

WALDBURGER, JENNIFER
SPIVACK, JILL
The Sleepeasy Solution: The Exhausted Parent's Guide to Getting Your Child to Sleep from Birth to Age 5.
HCI, April 2007

WEISSBLUTH, MARC.
Health Sleep Habits, Happy Child.
New York: Fawcett Books, 1999.

WEST, KIM
Good Night, Sleep Tight: Gentle Proven Solutions to Help Your Child Sleep Well and Wake Up Happy.
Vanguard Press, December 2009

INDEX

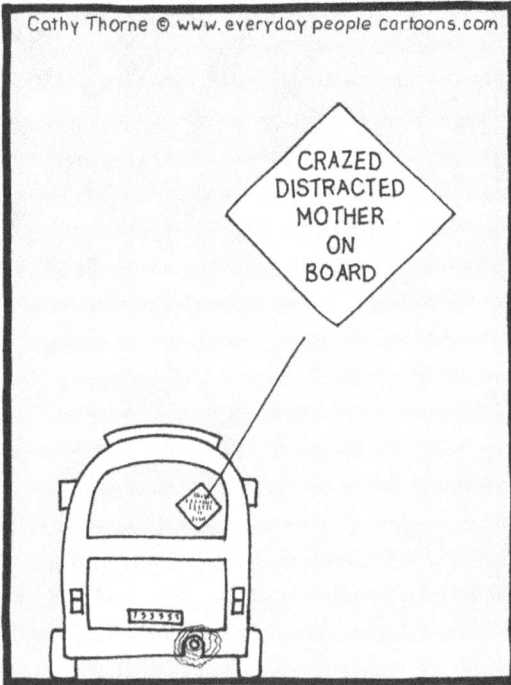

Cathy Thorne © www.everyday people cartoons.com

CRAZED DISTRACTED MOTHER ON BOARD

WHAT THE SIGN SHOULD SAY.

K
Kill Bill 44

L
Language 60, 70-71
Laughing 6, 8
Laughter 79
Laundry 7, 55, 78
Library 53, 71
Light 33-34, 39, 41-42, 45, 47, 49, 50-51, 54, 61, 65, 67, 77
Lullaby 66

M
Massage 33, 39, 46, 54, 57
Medicine 24, 28
Melatonin 50
Milk 20, 22, 29-30, 54,
Motion 39-40, 45, 61, 74-75, 81-82, 90
MP3 player 62, 63, 66, 71
Music 46, 50, 60-61, 62-63, 66, 71, 81, 85, 87

N
Nap 49, 76, 77, 79, 83, 85-86, 97
Nature 46, 48, 63-64, 66-67, 76, 81, 89
Newborn 4, 7, 15, 35-36, 76, 80, 90
Noise 58, 60-61, 62, 65, 67
Nose 25, 39, 57-58, 80

O
Onions 27
Oxygen 39, 41, 51, 64, 69, 79

P

ABOUT THE AUTHOR

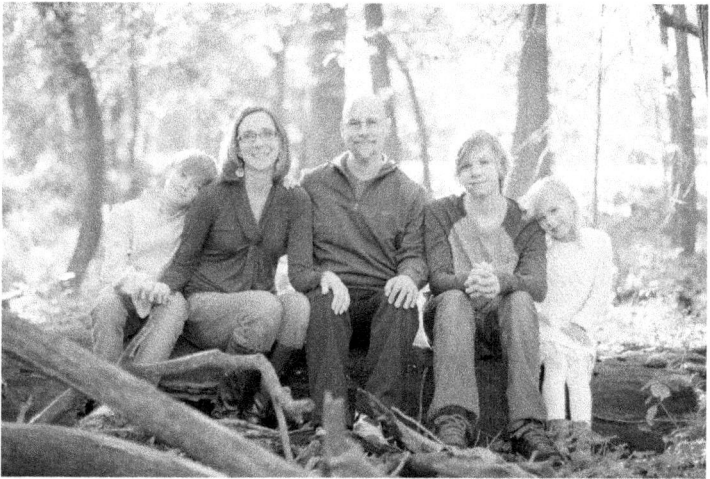

Kevin Mills has been a missionary, a market research analyst, a lawn boy, a receptionist and even performed as an energetic **Chuck E. Cheese** back in high school. (FYI, the costume isn't nearly as hot or stanky as you imagine. It's worse. *Much, much worse.*)

Kevin first became a Stay-at-Home Dad in 2002 when his first son **Kyler**, popped into the world. He's since been blessed with two more **K Clones**: **Kaleb** and **Kara**. While all three may act like insane, drunken monkeys at times, he loves them dearly as they have taught him how to slow down, have patience, and laugh at life more often. He and Kim have been married for almost 30 years and currently serve with **Mission**

Aviation Fellowship in **Papua, Indonesia**, teaching at **Hillcrest International School**.

In addition to his Dad duties, Kevin also oversees **Mills Creative Minds** as a product developer. His vision? To raise money for missionaries, churches and charities worldwide by giving away **70%** of the company's profits. Because there's more to life than fattening up a bank account and flashing bling. Much, much more.

Thank you for your support!

Kevin Mills